Dental
Instruments

EDITION
6

A POCKET GUIDE

P9-EEF-008

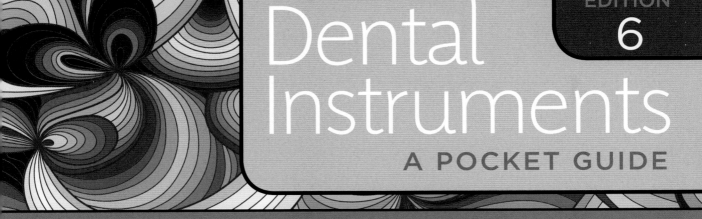

Dental Instruments

A POCKET GUIDE

EDITION 6

LINDA R. BARTOLOMUCCI BOYD, CDA, RDA, BA

Emeritus Professor, Registered Dental Assisting Program
Diablo Valley College
Pleasant Hill, California

ELSEVIER

ELSEVIER

3251 Riverport Lane
St. Louis, Missouri 63043

DENTAL INSTRUMENTS: A POCKET GUIDE, SIXTH EDITION

ISBN: 978-0-323474054

Notices

Knowledge and best practice in this field are constantly changing. As new research and experience broaden our understanding, changes in research methods, professional practices, or medical treatment may become necessary.

Practitioners and researchers must always rely on their own experience and knowledge in evaluating and using any information, methods, compounds, or experiments described herein. In using such information or methods they should be mindful of their own safety and the safety of others, including parties for whom they have a professional responsibility.

With respect to any drug or pharmaceutical products identified, readers are advised to check the most current information provided (i) on procedures featured or (ii) by the manufacturer of each product to be administered, to verify the recommended dose or formula, the method and duration of administration, and contraindications. It is the responsibility of practitioners, relying on their own experience and knowledge of their patients, to make diagnoses, to determine dosages and the best treatment for each individual patient, and to take all appropriate safety precautions.

To the fullest extent of the law, neither the Publisher nor the authors, contributors, or editors, assume any liability for any injury and/or damage to persons or property as a matter of products liability, negligence or otherwise, or from any use or operation of any methods, products, instructions, or ideas contained in the material herein.

ISBN: 978-0-323474054

Senior Content Strategist: Kristin Wilhelm
Content Development Specialist: Katie Gutierrez
Senior Content Development Specialist: Courtney Sprehe

Publishing Services Manager: Unni Deepthi
Senior Project Manager: Umarani Natarajan
Design Direction: Brian Salisbury

Printed in China

Last digit is the print number: 9   8   7   6   5   4   3   2   1

To Cathy Clarke . . . My appreciation for all of your expertise and dedication with your insight pertaining to innovative ideas for this edition as well as the past editions. Thank you!

To my college nieces and nephews, Raymond, Francesca, David, and Sophia, from whom I have learned the intricate way this current generation absorbs information and processes learning. Ti Amo!

Preface

It is with great pleasure that I present the sixth edition of *Dental Instruments: A Pocket Guide.*

Many new additions have been added to this text. First, the Sterilization Notes have more detailed information on how to process instruments. Second, many new photos were taken to enhance the working end as well as the entire instrument for clarity. Third, on the text page, many new photos are inserted to demonstrate the instrument "in use." Also, new technology equipment has been added, as well as new models of technology that already existed in the previous editions.

This text is designed to help dental students and practicing professionals master the identification and use of common and specialty dental instruments and equipment. Whereas certain chapters focus on the instruments used in all dental practices, such as components of the basic tray setup, the anesthetic syringe and its parts, evacuation devices, and so on, other chapters are designed around various routine dental procedures, such as the instruments used in hygiene, amalgam, and composite procedures. The dental specialty chapters include instruments used in prosthodontics, orthodontics, endodontics, and periodontics. Three chapters focus on oral surgery—one addresses the general surgical instruments used in oral and periodontal surgery, and the other two focus on surgical extractions and implants. The third focuses on periodontal instruments. Significant advances in detection of oral cancer equipment have been added to this text as well. There are also chapters devoted to dental material equipment.

Additionally, in keeping with the concept of total patient care, the chapter called "Vital Signs and Beyond" focuses on the equipment used to monitor patients for routine dental treatment as well as treatment of sedated patients. At the end of most chapters, there are examples of tray setups, enhancing the reader's ability to set up trays and use the instruments in the correct sequence, depending on the procedure.

In the 21st century, dentistry has certainly evolved with technology. It is more important than ever for students and clinicians to have an excellent understanding of the instruments and equipment they will encounter in practice. This sixth edition will help students and the clinicians stay current with the quickly changing technology of dentistry, as well as more detailed information on some instruments in the text pages. However, although basic dental instruments and equipment have remained relatively unchanged throughout the years, there have also been new advances that accommodate new technology in the dental field. These include, but are not limited to, the development of heat-resistant metals, synthetic material used for dental instruments, and new equipment. Examples can be seen in the special coatings available on some instruments, such as the titanium coating found on composite instruments that allow these instruments to be adapted to the different types of materials, as well as new designs of instruments.

I am confident that this text will help you to more easily learn the dental instruments, dental equipment, and tray setups that clinicians use in dental practices. It is imperative that all students begin their careers with a thorough knowledge of dental instruments and equipment and that they expand their knowledge throughout their careers. Certainly, this text will help you achieve these goals. I wish you all success in the field of dentistry. I know you will be a great asset to the dental profession!

Linda R. Bartolomucci Boyd

New to This Edition

- **Several new photos** in many chapters, including both a full-instrument view and close-up views to better see the working ends of the instruments to assist in easier identification
- **Additional "in use"** photos and illustrations of instruments and equipment to enhance the understanding of the function in specific procedures
- **Sequence of instruments** in the chapters have changed to give a better understanding of method of use for procedures.
- **Addition of new instruments and equipment,** including dental hygiene instruments and orthodontic equipment, as well as new technology on oral cancer detection.

FEATURES OF THIS TEXT

- **Flashcard format** makes it easy to quiz yourself on dental instruments and their uses.
- **More than 700 high-quality photographs and illustrations** enhance your ability to quickly and accurately identify dental instruments.

- Convenient **spiral-bound design** helps you easily access key information at a glance as well as use the pages as a **flash card technique** for studying.
- **Clear, consistent organization** helps you master basic instruments before introducing more complicated instruments.
- **Tray setups** (Note: The tray setups usually only have an example of instruments for the designated procedure; they do not include any axillary items needed for that particular procedure, such as cotton rolls or 2 × 2 gauze.)

Each written page has information on each individual instrument including:

- Name of the instrument
- Main function of the instrument
- Characteristics of the instrument
- Practice Note
- Sterilization Note
- In addition to the Sterilization Note on each written page, it should be noted that instruments and items used during dental procedures are categorized as critical, semicritical, or noncritical. Below are excerpts from the *Guidelines for Infection Control in Dental Health-Care Settings—2003* that explain the categories.

- "Patient-care items (dental instruments, devices, and equipment) are categorized as critical, semicritical, or noncritical, depending on the potential risk for infection associated with their intended use. . . . Critical items used to penetrate soft tissue or bone have the greatest risk of transmitting infection and should be sterilized by heat. Semicritical items touch mucous membranes or nonintact skin and have a lower risk of transmission; because the majority of semicritical items in dentistry are heat-tolerant, they also should be sterilized by using heat. If a semicritical item is heat-sensitive, it should, at a minimum, be processed with high-level disinfection. . . .
- "Noncritical patient-care items pose the least risk of transmission of infection, contacting only intact skin, which can serve as an effective barrier to microorganisms. In the majority of cases, cleaning, or if visibly soiled, cleaning followed by disinfection with an EPA-registered hospital disinfectant is adequate. When the item is visibly contaminated with blood or OPIM, an EPA-registered hospital disinfectant with a tuberculocidal claim (i.e., intermediate-level disinfectant) should be used. . . . Cleaning or disinfection of certain noncritical patient-care items can be difficult or damage the surfaces; therefore, use of disposable barrier protection of these surfaces might be a preferred alternative."
- For detailed information regarding guidelines for infection control in a dental setting please refer to *Guidelines for Infection Control in Dental Health-Care Settings—2003* at http://www.cdc.gov/mmwr/index.html.

EVOLVE

For the Student ▸ Chapter Quizzes • Drag-and-Drop Tray Setup Exercises • Tray Setup Quizzes

For the Instructor ▸ Image Collection for Power Point Presentation and Testing • Test Bank

Acknowledgements

My deepest appreciation is to acknowledge all of my colleagues, dentist affiliations, professors, and my dearest family and friends for all of their insight, support, love, and prayers during the writing of this sixth edition. Of course, I value each and every student because their zest and enthusiasm for learning give me such encouragement to write a text that enhances their desire to learn.

Two people have played an incredible role in making this text such a great learning tool with the availability of the instruments and the creative skill in photography. First and foremost, I have the greatest respect for Jeff McMillian in his ability to photograph dental instruments. Jeff's artistic ability and incredible photography skills have enhanced this text with clearer and more precise photographs, especially the close-up working ends of dental instruments and the all-new photographs of the instruments "in use." Second, these photographs would not be possible without Andrew Hartzell, president of G. Hartzell & Son, Inc., who allowed me to borrow most of the instruments to photograph. Thank you, Andy!

I am absolutely grateful to Katie Gutierrez, content development specialist, and to Courtney Sprehe, senior content development specialist, for their development of the sixth edition of this text. Courtney's vision and mine have remained the same from the second edition to now the sixth. Kristin Wilhelm, I thank you for your expertise as editor in overseeing and publishing this sixth edition.

I continue to express my thanks to **Joyce M. Litch, RDH, DDS, MSD,** for her expertise as a consultant to the book, who assisted in developing the periodontal and hygiene chapters. I thank you for always being there for me! **Ann Marie Gorczyca, DMD, MPH, MS,** you are amazing in your enthusiasm in encouraging me to always follow my passion. Thank you, for your words of praise and encouragement in the ongoing process of publishing and your expertise in knowledge of orthodontics and beyond. The bur chapter would not be as comprehensive without the consultation from **Wayne Joseph, DDS.** His insight into this chapter has been appreciated from the first edition to the sixth.

I would like to express my deepest gratitude to **Cathy Clarke, RDA, CDA, BA,** to whom this book is dedicated, who spent numerous hours and days as a consultant to many aspects of this text. Thank you for always being available to answer my questions at any time. A very special thank you to Paul Charles Hans, BS, MBA, an author himself, for his ability in keeping my focus in the process of the photography as well as the creative technical writing of this text. Your love, support, and encouragement mean more to me than I can express.

I could not have written this sixth edition without the love, support, and prayers from my family: my sons, Michael and Matthew, who always gave me a nudge of encouragement; my cousin Elaine Strizzi, for her gentle and loving ways of support; and my brother and sister-in-law, Ray and Meri, for the nourishment of my body and soul during this process. Also, the concept my parents taught me, "To honor the dream inside of me," constantly resonates in my mind. Last, but certainly not least, are the wonderful, refreshing moments with my grandchildren, Christian, Collin, Liberty Rae, Alexis, Jaxson, and Maxwell, who teach me the simplicity, enthusiasm, and zest for learning that encourages my writing. Ti Amo!

Linda R. Bartolomucci Boyd
For information about the author or to ask questions about the text, please contact lrboyd47@yahoo.com.

Contents

Photo/Illustration Credits

Mirion Technologies, Dosimetry Service Division:
p. 680 [www.mirion.com]

Obtura Spartan Endodontics: p. 316 [www.obtura.com]

Patterson Dental Co. Inc.: p. 408 (left)
[www.pattersondental.com]

Paradise Dental Technologies (PDT), Inc.: p. 358
[www.pdtdental.com]

Porter Instruments Division, Parker Hannifin Corp: pp.
54 (left), 56 [www.porterinstrument.com]

Practicon Inc.: pp. 54 (right), 660 [www.practicon.com]

Premier Dental: pp. 292, 294, 296 [www.premusa.com]

SciCan Inc. (STATIM G4): p. 616 [www.scican.com]

Tatum Surgical: p. 570 [www.tatumsurgical.com]

Vita North America, Inc.: pp. 258, 259
[www.vitanorthamerica.com]

Wayne Metal Products: p. 618
[www.waynemetalproductsinc.com]

Whip Mix Corporation: pp. 256, 257, 650, 652
[www.whipmix.com]

Zest Dental Solutions: p. 104 [www.zestanchors.com]

Zewa Inc.: p. 726 [www.zewa.com]

Hu-Friedy Mfg. Co., LLC: pp. 48 (right), 174,
176, 178, 180, 300, 362, 363, 364, 366, 368, 370,
374, 592, 594, 596, 598, 600, 602, 604, 608, 658,
659 [www.hu-friedy.com]

i-CAT: p. 716 [www.i-cat.com]

Innoden, LLC (BIOX portable x-ray unit): p. 708
[www.innoden.com]

Isolite Systems: pp. 66–67 [www.isolitesystems.com]

Ivoclar Vivadent: p. 202 (left)
[www.ivoclarvivadent.com]

Kavo Kerr: pp. 72 (left), 86, 88, 392, 246, 247,
282, 304, 384, 385, 630, 634, 638, 647, 678, 682
[www.kavokerrgroup.com]

Kerr Corporation, on behalf of Pentron Clinical Technologies, LLC: pp. 644, 646
[www.pentron.com]

LED Dental Inc.: p. 718 [www.leddental.com]

Midmark Corp.: pp. 612, 614 [www.midmark.com]

ZOLL Medical Corporation: p. 734 [www.zoll.com]

Photo/Illustration Credits (Books)

Aschheim KW: Esthetic dentistry: a clinical approach to techniques and materials, ed 3, St. Louis, 2015, Mosby—illustration on page 391

Baum L, Phillips RW, Lund MR: Textbook of operative dentistry, ed 3, Philadelphia, 1995, Saunders—illustrations on pages 5, 16 (right), 23, 35, 121, 123, 125, 127, 169, 171

Bird DL, Robinson DS: Torres and Ehrlich modern dental assisting, ed 8, St. Louis, 2005, Saunders—illustrations on pages 205, 207

Bird DL, Robinson DS: Torres and Ehrlich modern dental assisting, ed 9, St. Louis, 2009, Saunders—illustration on page 674

Bird DL, Robinson DS: Modern dental assisting, ed 11, St. Louis, 2015, Elsevier—illustrations on pages 131, 133, 261

Bird DL, Robinson DS: Modern dental assisting, ed 12, St. Louis, 2018, Elsevier—illustrations on pages 3, 7, 63, 65, 97, 175, 190, 202, 209, 219, 243, 383, 585, 587, 597, 625, 627, 631, 642, 649, 651, 657, 666, 687, 695, 712

Convissar RA: Principles and practice of laser dentistry, ed 2, St. Louis, 2016, Mosby—illustration on page 393

Darby ML, Walsh M: Dental hygiene: theory and practice, ed 4, St. Louis, 2015, Saunders—illustrations on pages 55 (Courtesy Dr. Mark Dellinges), 163, 183, 193, 197, 199, 213, 263

Dean JA, Avery DR, McDonald RE: McDonald and Avery dentistry for the child and adolescent, ed 10, St. Louis, 2016, Elsevier—illustrations on pages 265, 483

Fairchild SL: Pierson and Fairchild's principles and techniques of patient care, ed 5, St. Louis, 2013, Saunders—illustration on page 735

Harrick CD, Eakle WS, Bird WF: Dental materials: clinical applications for dental assistants and dental hygienists, St. Louis, 2003, Saunders—illustration on page 354

Harrick CD, Eakle WS, Bird WF: Dental materials: clinical applications for dental assistants and dental hygienists, ed 3, St. Louis, 2016, Elsevier—illustrations on pages 153, 245, 249, 641, 643, 659

Heymann HO, Swift EJ, Ritter AV: Sturdevant's art and science of operative dentistry, ed 6, St. Louis, 2013, Mosby—illustration on page 31

Hupp JR, Ellis E, Tucker MR: Contemporary oral and maxillofacial surgery, ed 6, St. Louis, 2014, Mosby—illustrations on pages 495, 535, 555, 606, 681

Iannucci J, Howerton LJ: Dental radiography: principles and techniques, ed 5, St. Louis, 2017, Elsevier—illustrations on pages 688, 692 (adapted)

Malamed SF: Handbook of local anesthesia, ed 6, St. Louis, 2013, Mosby—illustration on page 45

Malamed SF: Sedation: a guide to patient management, ed 5, St. Louis, 2010, Mosby—illustration on page 481

Fehrenbach MJ, Herring SW: Illustrated anatomy of the head and neck, ed 5, St. Louis, 2017, Elsevier—illustration on page 39 (Photo courtesy Margaret Fehrenbach)

Freedman G: Contemporary esthetic dentistry, St. Louis, 2012, Mosby—illustration on page 388

Garg AK: Implant dentistry, ed 2, St. Louis, 2010, Mosby—illustration on page 549

Graber TM, Vanarsdall RL, Vig KWL: Orthodontics: current principles and techniques, ed 4, St. Louis, 2006, Mosby—illustration on page 418

Graber LW, Vanarsdall RL, Vig KWL, et al: Orthodontics: current principles and techniques, ed 6, St. Louis, 2017, Elsevier—illustration on page 459

Gutmann JL, Lovdahl PE: Problem solving in endodontics: prevention, identification and management, ed 5, St. Louis, 2011, Mosby—illustrations on pages 485, 497

Hargreaves KM, Berman LH: Cohen's pathways of the pulp, Expert Consult, ed 11, St. Louis, 2016, Elsevier—illustrations on pages 287, 313, 317, 321

Newman MG, Takei H, Klokkevold PR, Carranza FA: Carranza's clinical periodontology, ed 11, St. Louis, 2012, Saunders—illustrations on pages 343, 345, 372, 373, 511, 517

Papadopoulos MA, Tarawneh F: The use of miniscrew implants for temporary skeletal anchorage in orthodontics: a comprehensive review. *Oral Surgery, Oral Medicine, Oral* Pathology, *Oral Radiology, and Endodontology*, 103(5): e6-e15, 2007—illustration on page 468 (left)

Perry DA, Beemsterboer PL: Periodontology for the dental hygienist, ed 4, St. Louis, 2014, Saunders—illustrations on pages 355, 513, 572

Proctor DB, Young-Adams AP: Kinn's the medical assistant: an applied learning approach, ed 13, St. Louis, 2017, Elsevier—illustrations on pages 724, 729

Proffit WR, Fields HW, Sarver DM: Contemporary orthodontics, ed 5, St. Louis, 2013, Mosby—illustrations on pages 405, 407, 419, 439, 441, 461

Robinson DS, Bird DL: Essentials of dental assisting, ed 5, St. Louis, 2013, Saunders—illustration on page 118

Rose LF, Mealey BL, Genco RJ, Cohen W: Periodontics: medicine, surgery and implants, St. Louis, 2004, Mosby—illustrations on pages 503, 519

Rosenstiel SF, Land MF, Fujimoto J: Contemporary fixed prosthodontics, ed 4, St. Louis, 2006, Mosby—illustration on page 155

Rosenstiel SF, Land MF, Fujimoto J: Contemporary fixed prosthodontics, ed 5, St. Louis, 2016, Elsevier—illustrations on pages 137, 143, 155, 273, 307, 315

Singh PP, Cranin AN: Atlas of oral implantology, ed 3, St. Louis, 2010, Mosby—illustrations on pages 293, 489, 491, 545

White SC, Pharoah MJ: Oral radiology: principles and interpretation, ed 7, St. Louis, 2014, Mosby—illustration on page 684 (adapted)

Basic Dental Instruments

Mouth Mirror

Functions ▶
To provide indirect vision
To retract lips, cheeks, and tongue
To reflect light into the mouth

Characteristics ▶
1 Front surface mirrors—Accurate, distortion-free image
2 Double-sided mirrors—Used to retract tongue or cheek and view intraoral cavity simultaneously
Flat surface mirrors—Used in disposable mirrors
Concave mirrors—Magnify image
Range of sizes
Commonly used sizes: no. 4 and no. 5; refer to diameter of mirror
Single ended
Different mirror handles available (see p. 8)

Practice Notes ▶
Mouth Mirror is used on most tray setups.

Sterilization Notes ▶
Mouth Mirror must be precleaned, either, placed in a sterilizing pouch with an internal process indicator, sealed, then sterilized OR wrapped with an internal process indicator inside and secured on the outside with process indicator tape, then sterilized. Verify appropriate color change has been achieved in external process indicator immediately after removal from sterilizer then check internal process indicator before treatment. Refer to state regulations for any additional state requirements.

Explorers

Function ▶ To examine teeth for decay (caries), calculus, furcations, or other abnormalities

Characteristics ▶ Pointed tips; sharp, thin, flexible
Single or double ended

- Double-ended models—May have the same style on working ends or different styles of working ends; may also have explorer on one end and periodontal probe on the other end (for periodontal probe, see Chapter 16).

Variety of sizes and types:

1. Orban
2. Pigtail
3. Shepherd's hook

Practice Notes ▶ Explorer is used on most tray setups.

Sterilization Notes ▶ Explorer must be precleaned, either, placed in a sterilizing pouch with an internal process indicator, sealed, then sterilized OR wrapped with an internal process indicator inside and secured on the outside with process indicator tape, then sterilized. Verify appropriate color change has been achieved in external process indicator immediately after removal from sterilizer then check internal process indicator before treatment. Refer to state regulations for any additional state requirements.

■INSTRUMENT Cotton Forceps (Pliers)

Function ▶ To grasp or transfer items and/or material into and out of the oral cavity

Characteristics ▶ Plain or serrated tips
Pointed or rounded tips
Thin or thick tips
Locking forceps (see Chapter 11)
Range of sizes available

Practice Notes ▶ Cotton Forceps is used on most tray setups.

Sterilization Notes ▶ Cotton Forceps must be precleaned, either, placed in a sterilizing pouch with an internal process indicator, sealed, then sterilized OR wrapped with an internal process indicator inside and secured on the outside with process indicator tape, then sterilized. Verify appropriate color change has been achieved in external process indicator immediately after removal from sterilizer then check internal process indicator before treatment. Refer to state regulations for any additional state requirements.

Instrument Handles

Function ▶ To hold (grasp) instrument

Characteristics ▶ Single or double ended
Removable working ends (replaceable and interchangeable) attach to handle
Examples: Mouth mirror, scaler

Nonremovable working ends also available (commonly used)
Larger diameter models—Help lighten grasp and maximize control
Alternating diameter models—Lessen stress associated with carpal tunnel syndrome
Lighter weight models—Minimize fatigue
Variety of sizes, styles, and textures:

1 Small, round ¼-inch stainless steel
2 Standard, hollow ⁵⁄₁₆-inch stainless steel
3 Lightweight, ⅜-inch slip-resistant pattern
4 Satin steel model—Lightweight, ergonomically designed

Sterilization Notes ▶ Instrument Handles must be precleaned, either, placed in a sterilizing pouch with an internal process indicator, sealed, then sterilized OR wrapped with an internal process indicator inside and secured on the outside with process indicator tape, then sterilized. Verify appropriate color change has been achieved in external process indicator immediately after removal from sterilizer then check internal process indicator before treatment. Refer to state regulations for any additional state requirements.

Basic

FROM TOP TO BOTTOM

Mouth mirror, explorer (pigtail explorer pictured), cotton forceps (example of color-coded instruments in a cassette)

Practice Notes ▶ Basic Setup is found on almost all dental tray setups.

Sterilization Notes ▶ Basic Setup instruments with cassette must be precleaned, either, placed in a sterilizing pouch with an internal process indicator, sealed, then sterilized OR wrapped with an internal process indicator inside and secured on the outside with process indicator tape, then sterilized. Verify appropriate color change has been achieved in external process indicator immediately after removal from sterilizer then check internal process indicator before treatment. Refer to state regulations for any additional state requirements.

Enamel-Cutting Instruments

Parts of an Instrument

1 **Handle ▶** Grasping end of instrument
Variety of sizes and styles
Handle styles (refer to pp. 8 & 9)

2 **Shank ▶** Connects handle to working end of instrument
May be straight or may have one or more angles to accommodate specific areas of the
mouth

3 **Working End ▶** May have cutting edge, blade, bevel, point, nib, or beaks

Three-Numbered Instrument*

Function ▶ Numbers on handle indicate width, length, and angle of blade.

1 Indicates width of blade in tenths of millimeters
Example: 20 indicates a width of 2 mm

2 Indicates length of blade in millimeters
Example: 8 indicates a length of 8 mm

3 Indicates angle of blade from long axis of shaft
Example: 12 indicates an angle of 12 degrees

The designation for the instrument described above is 20-8-12; the number of instrument size is indicated on the handle.
Examples of three-numbered instruments: Enamel, Hatchet, Enamel, Hoe, Wedelstaedt

*The instrument number formula was designed by Dr. G.V. Black, Northwestern University.

Four-Numbered Instrument*

Function ► Numbers on handle indicate width of blade, angle of cutting edge, length of blade, and angle of blade.

1 Indicates width of blade in tenths of millimeters
Example: 20 indicates a width of 2 mm

2 Indicates angle of cutting edge of blade in relation to handle
Example: 95 indicates a cutting edge angle of 95 degrees

3 Indicates length of blade in millimeters
Example: 8 indicates a length of 8 mm

4 Indicates angle of blade from long axis of shaft
Example: 12 indicates a blade angle of 12 degrees

The designation for the instrument described above is 20-95-8-12; The number of instrument size is indicated on the handle.
Examples of four-numbered instruments: Angle Former, Gingival Margin Trimmers—Mesial and Distal

*The instrument number formula was designed by Dr. G.V. Black, Northwestern University.

■INSTRUMENT Enamel Hatchet

Functions ▶ To cut, clean, and smooth walls in cavity preparation
To remove enamel not supported by dentin

Characteristics ▶ Used with push motion
Cutting edge on same plane as handle
Single or double ended
Is a three-numbered instrument
Examples of instrument numbers:

20-9-14
15-8-14
15-8-12

Practice Notes ▶ Enamel Hatchet is used on restorative tray setups.

Sterilization Notes ▶ Enamel Hatchet must be precleaned, either, placed in
a sterilizing pouch with an internal process indicator,
sealed, then sterilized OR wrapped with an internal process indicator inside and secured
on the outside with process indicator tape, then sterilized. Verify appropriate color change
has been achieved in external process indicator immediately after removal from sterilizer
then check internal process indicator before treatment. Refer to state regulations for any
additional state requirements.

■INSTRUMENT Enamel Hoe

Function ▶ To clean and smooth floor and walls in cavity preparation

Characteristics ▶ Used with pulling motion
Cutting edge or blade nearly perpendicular to handle
Is a three-numbered instrument
Examples of instrument numbers:

10-4-8
10-4-14

Practice Notes ▶ Enamel Hoe is used on restorative tray setups.

Sterilization Notes ▶ Enamel Hoe must be precleaned, either, placed in a
sterilizing pouch with an internal process indicator, sealed,
then sterilized OR wrapped with an internal process indicator
inside and secured on the outside with process indicator
tape, then sterilized. Verify appropriate color change has been achieved in external process
indicator immediately after removal from sterilizer then check internal process indicator
before treatment. Refer to state regulations for any additional state requirements.

Straight Chisel

Function ▶ To plane and cleave enamel in cavity preparation

Characteristics ▶ Used with push motion
Single-bevel cutting edge
Single or double ended

Examples of instrument numbers:

15
20

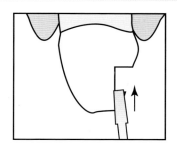

Practice Notes ▶ Straight Chisel is used on restorative tray setups.

Sterilization Notes ▶ Straight Chisel must be precleaned, either, placed in a sterilizing pouch with an internal process indicator, sealed, then sterilized OR wrapped with an internal process indicator inside and secured on the outside with process indicator tape, then sterilized. Verify appropriate color change has been achieved in external process indicator immediately after removal from sterilizer then check internal process indicator before treatment. Refer to state regulations for any additional state requirements.

Wedelstaedt Chisel

Function ▶ To plane and cleave enamel in cavity preparation

Characteristics ▶ Used with push motion
Curved blade on working end
Single-bevel cutting edge
Single or double ended
Is a three-numbered instrument

Examples of instrument numbers:

15-15-3
11.5-15-3

Practice Notes ▶ Wedelstaedt Chisel is used on restorative tray setups.

Sterilization Notes ▶ Wedelstaedt Chisel must be precleaned, either, placed in a
sterilizing pouch with an internal process indicator, sealed, then
sterilized OR wrapped with an internal process indicator inside
and secured on the outside with process indicator tape, then
sterilized. Verify appropriate color change has been achieved in external process indicator
immediately after removal from sterilizer then check internal process indicator before
treatment. Refer to state regulations for any additional state requirements.

▪INSTRUMENT Binangle Chisel

Function ▸ To plane and cleave enamel in cavity preparation

Characteristics ▸ Used with push motion
Two angles in the shank
Single or double ended
Is an example of three-numbered instrument

Examples of instrument numbers:

20-9-8
15-8-8

Practice Notes ▸ Binangle Chisel is used on restorative tray setups.

Sterilization Notes ▸ Binangle Chisel must be precleaned, either, placed in
a sterilizing pouch with an internal process indicator, sealed, then sterilized OR wrapped
with an internal process indicator inside and secured on the outside with process indicator
tape, then sterilized. Verify appropriate color change has been achieved in external process
indicator immediately after removal from sterilizer then check internal process indicator
before treatment. Refer to state regulations for any additional state requirements.

Angle Former

Function ▶ To accentuate line and point angles in internal outline and retention in cavity preparation

Characteristics ▶ Cutting edge at an angle
Single or double ended
Is a four-numbered instrument

Examples of instrument numbers:

12-80-5-8
9-80-4-8

Practice Notes ▶ Angle Former is used on restorative tray setups.

Sterilization Notes ▶ Angle Former must be precleaned, either, placed in a
sterilizing pouch with an internal process indicator, sealed, then sterilized OR wrapped
with an internal process indicator inside and secured on the outside with process indicator
tape, then sterilized. Verify appropriate color change has been achieved in external process
indicator immediately after removal from sterilizer then check internal process indicator
before treatment. Refer to state regulations for any additional state requirements.

Gingival Margin Trimmer—Mesial and Distal

Function ▸ To bevel cervical walls of mesial and distal retention areas

Characteristics ▸

1 Mesial: To create bevels on the mesial cervical margin of the preparation
2 Distal: To create bevels on the distal cervical margin of the preparation

Curved blade
Cutting edge at angle to blade
Double ended (one end curves to the right; the other to the left)
Is a four-numbered instrument

Examples of instrument numbers:

Mesial: 13-80-8-14 or 15-80-8-12
Distal: 13-95-8-14 or 15-95-8-12

Practice Notes ▸ Gingival Margin Trimmer is used on restorative tray setups.
Gingival Margin Trimmer is placed on tray setups in pairs: mesial and distal.
Refer to the amalgam tray setup in Chapter 8.

Sterilization Notes ▸ Gingival Margin Trimmer must be precleaned, either, placed in a sterilizing pouch with an internal process indicator, sealed, then sterilized OR wrapped with an internal process indicator inside and secured on the outside with process indicator tape, then sterilized. Verify appropriate color change has been achieved in external process indicator immediately after removal from sterilizer then check internal process indicator before treatment. Refer to state regulations for any additional state requirements.

Spoon Excavators

Function ▶ To remove carious dentin
Secondary functions:
To remove temporary crowns
To remove temporary cement in temporary restoration
To remove permanent crown during try-in

Characteristics ▶ Concave design, spoon-shaped with cutting edge

Range of sizes:

1 Large—Curved blade—also referred to as Black Spoon
2 Small—Round blade

Single or double ended

Practice Notes ▶ Spoon Excavator is used on restorative tray setups.
Refer to the amalgam tray setup (see Chapter 8), composite tray setups (see Chapter 9), and crown and bridge restorative tray setups (see Chapter 10).

Sterilization Notes ▶ Spoon Excavator must be precleaned, either, placed in a sterilizing pouch with an internal process indicator, sealed, then sterilized OR wrapped with an internal process indicator inside and secured on the outside with process indicator tape, then sterilized. Verify appropriate color change has been achieved in external process indicator immediately after removal from sterilizer then check internal process indicator before treatment. Refer to state regulations for any additional state requirements.

Local Anesthetic Syringe/ Components and Nitrous Oxide Sedation

Anesthetic Aspirating Syringe

Function ▶ To administer a local anesthetic

Characteristics ▶ Parts:

1 Threaded tip **2** Harpoon
3 Piston rod **4** Barrel of syringe
5 Finger grip **6** Finger bar
7 Thumb ring **8** Syringe assembled with needle
and anesthetic cartridge

Practice Notes ▶ Syringes with harpoons are considered aspirating syringes.
Disposable syringes equipped with needles and preloaded with anesthetic are available.
Anesthetic Aspirating Syringe is used on most tray setups.

Sterilization Notes ▶ Anesthetic Aspirating Syringe must be precleaned, either, placed in a sterilizing pouch with an internal process indicator, sealed, then sterilized OR wrapped with an internal process indicator inside and secured on the outside with process indicator tape, then sterilized. Verify appropriate color change has been achieved in external process indicator immediately after removal from sterilizer then check internal process indicator before treatment. Refer to state regulations for any additional state requirements. Disposable preloaded syringes with needle must be disposed of in a sharps container. Anesthetic cartridge and needle must be disposed of in a sharps container. Refer to local and state recommendations for disposal of anesthetic cartridge.

Short Needle

Function ▶ To administer anesthetic by infiltration injection on maxillary arch

Characteristics ▶ Parts:

1. Cartridge end of needle
2. Needle hub
3. Injection end of needle
4. Lumen of the needle
5. Bevel of the needle
6. Protective cap
7. Seal on cap
8. Needle guard

1 inch long for infiltration injection
1. End of needle inserts into the anesthetic cartridge
4. Anesthetic solution is ejected through the lumen of the needle
Variety of gauges:

- Gauge number—Identifies diameter (thickness) of needle
- Larger gauge number—Indicates thinner needle (e.g., 30 gauge is thinner than 25 gauge)

Practice Notes ▶ Local anesthetic syringe setup is used on most tray setups

Sterilization Notes ▶ Short Needle must be disposed of in a sharps container. Single use only.

Long Needle

Function ▶ To administer anesthetic by block injection on mandibular arch

Characteristics ▶ Parts:

1	Cartridge end of needle	**2**	Needle hub
3	Injection end of needle	**4**	Lumen of the needle
5	Bevel of the needle	**6**	Protective cap
7	Seal on cap	**8**	Needle guard

$1\frac{5}{8}$ inches long for block injection

1 End of needle inserts into the anesthetic cartridge
4 Anesthetic solution is ejected through the lumen of the needle
Variety of gauges:

- Gauge number—Identifies diameter (thickness) of needle
- Larger gauge number—Indicates thinner needle (e.g., 30 gauge is thinner than 25 gauge)

Practice Notes ▶ Local anesthetic syringe setup is used on most tray setups.

Sterilization Notes ▶ Long Needle must be disposed of in a sharps container. Single use only.

Anesthetic Cartridge

Function ▶ To hold liquid anesthetic for local injection in the oral cavity

Characteristics ▶ Parts:

1 Rubber diaphragm—Syringe needle is inserted into the diaphragm to penetrate into the cartridge.

2 Aluminum cap holds the rubber diaphragm in place.

3 Glass cartridge (also referred to as a carpule)

4 Indicates type of anesthesia

5 Color-coded band indicating type of anesthetic (required by the American Dental Association, June 2003)

6 Silicon rubber plunger—Harpoon of syringe inserts into silicon rubber plunger.

Composition of solution in cartridge—Contains 1.7 to 1.8 mL of anesthetic solution
Plunger slightly indented from rim of glass

Practice Notes ▶ Type of anesthetic used depends on patient's health history and dental procedure performed. Local anesthetic syringe setup is used on most tray setups.

Sterilization Notes ▶ Anesthetic Cartridge must be disposed of in a sharps container. Refer to local and state recommendations for disposal of cartridge. Single use only.

■INSTRUMENT Anesthetic Cartridges/Blister Packs

Function ▶ To hold liquid anesthetic for injection

Characteristics ▶ Several types of anesthetic solutions available
Each cartridge is labeled.
Color code system on cartridge—Identifies type of anesthetic (required by the American Dental Association, June 2003). Color band on each cartridge indicates type of anesthetic solution.
Type of anesthetic used depends on patient's health history and dental procedure performed:

1. Anesthetic is available without a vasoconstrictor.
2. Ratio of epinephrine: the lower the second number, the higher the percentage of vasoconstrictor. Information printed on cartridge. Example of common anesthetic for routine dental procedures 1:100,000.
3. Longer lasting anesthetic has a higher percentage of vasoconstrictor. Example: 1:50,000.

Practice Notes ▶ Remove each cartridge from blister pack as needed for each procedure and place cartridge on tray setup.
Local anesthetic syringe setup is used on most tray setups.

Sterilization Notes ▶ Anesthetic Cartridge must be disposed of in a sharps container. Refer to local and state recommendations for disposal of cartridge. Each anesthetic cartridge for single use only.

▪INSTRUMENT Recapping Device

Function ▶ To hold needle sheath for one-hand recapping after injection

Characteristics ▶
1 Jenker—Low center of gravity for stability in recapping
2 Needle cap holder attached to cassette

Helps prevent needle stick accidents
Different styles of needle stick protectors available

Practice Notes ▶ Needle Stick Protector is used on most tray setups.
Scoop Technique Procedure—Recap needle by scooping end of
needle into needle guard (not shown).

Sterilization Notes ▶ Needle Stick Protector—Jenker or needle cap holder must be
precleaned, either, placed in a sterilizing pouch with an internal process
indicator, sealed, then sterilized OR wrapped with an internal process
indicator inside and secured on the outside with process indicator tape,
then sterilized. Verify appropriate color change has been achieved in
external process indicator immediately after removal from sterilizer
then check internal process indicator before treatment. Refer to state regulations for any
additional state requirements. Disposable preloaded syringes with needle must be disposed
of in a sharps container. Anesthetic cartridge and needle must be disposed of in a sharps
container. Refer to local and state recommendations for disposal of anesthetic cartridge.

Computer-Controlled Local Anesthetic Delivery System (The Wand/STA Single Tooth Anesthesia System)

Functions ▶
To administer a local anesthetic
To improve ergonomics and precision of dental anesthetic delivery

Characteristics ▶
Lightweight wand handpiece held in a penlike grip.
Presterilized bonded handpiece (not a traditional dental syringe)
Foot-activated control delivers local anesthetic.
Computer controls available flow rates of local anesthetic, making them consistent.
Aspiration test can be activated at any time by releasing the pressure cycle on the foot rheostat.
Can be used for all dental injections and intraligamentary (PDL) injection

Practice Notes ▶
The operator focuses on needle insertion and positioning while the motor in the device administers the drug at a preprogrammed rate of flow.
Increased tactile control and ergonomics decreases patient discomfort.

Sterilization Notes ▶
Anesthetic cartridge must be disposed of in a biohazard container.
Refer to local and state recommendations for disposal of cartridge. Single use only. Needle must be disposed of in a sharps container. Single use only. Tubing must be disposed of in garbage. One time use only. Refer to manufacturer's recommendation for disinfection of unit.

▪INSTRUMENT Nitrous Oxide and Analgesic Tanks

Function ▶ To use as an analgesic to relax patients for dental procedures
To be inhaled through a mask placed over the nose

Characteristic ▶
1 Blue tank is N_2O
2 Green tank is O_2

Nitrous oxide is a chemical compound with the formula N_2O. It is an oxide of nitrogen.
Room temperature, N_2O is a colorless, nonflammable gas, with a slightly sweet odor and taste
Nose piece has tubing attached to a scavenger system that evacuates excess N_2O that patient does not breath.

Practice Notes ▶ Nitrous oxide is used for apprehensive patients for all types of dental procedures.
Oxygen must be given to patient before dismissing from the dental chair.
Fail-safe system:
All N_2O and O_2 systems used in dentistry have a fail-safe system.
Sufficient amount of O_2 gas must be present in the tank while system is functioning or the system will shut down.

Sterilization Notes ▶ Nitrous Oxide Tanks—refer to manufacturer's recommendation for disinfection.

Nitrous Oxide Nasal Mask

Functions ▸ To place mask over the patient's nose for the delivery of N_2O

To evacuate excess N_2O that is not breathed in by the patient

Characteristics ▸
1 Tubing for N_2O
2 Tubing for scavenger system to evacuate excess N_2O
3 Disposable masks available in different scents

Different size masks available for children and adults.

Practice Notes ▸ Gauze is placed under mask for patient comfort. N_2O is used for apprehensive patients for all types of dental procedures.

Oxygen must be given to the patient before dismissing the patient from the dental chair.

Sterilization Notes ▸ N_2O Masks refer to manufacturer's recommendation for sterilization. Disposable masks single use only. Dispose of in the garbage.

▪INSTRUMENT **Nitrous Oxide and Oxygen Flowmeters**

Function ▶ To monitor the N_2O and O_2 that is administered to the patient

Characteristics ▶
1. % N_2O adjustment knob: Controls the % of N_2O
2. Total flow adjustment knob: Controls the combined flow of O_2 and N_2O or O_2 flow only when the % of N_2O knob is set to zero
3. Digital display readout of N_2O and O_2 using knobs for adjustment of gas flow.

Tubing from the tanks go to flowmeters and tubing from flowmeters go to the face mask that delivers the gases to the patient.

All masks have tubing attached to a scavenger system: An appropriate evacuation/HVE system that evacuates the excess gas that the patient does not inhale.

Practice Notes ▶ N_2O is used for apprehensive patients for all types of dental procedures.
Oxygen must be given to the patient before dismissing from the dental chair.

Sterilization Notes ▶ Flowmeters refer to manufacturer's recommendation for disinfection.

Local Anesthetic Syringe

From Left to Right ▶ Anesthetic aspirating syringe, long needle, short needle, anesthetic cartridges, needle stick protector (Jenker) (top right), individually packed topical anesthetic (bottom right)

Practice Notes ▶ Local Anesthetic Syringe setup is found on most tray setups.

Sterilization Notes ▶ Anesthetic Syringe and Needle Stick Protector must be precleaned, either, placed in a sterilizing pouch with an internal process indicator, sealed, then sterilized OR wrapped with an internal process indicator inside and secured on the outside with process indicator tape, then sterilized. Verify appropriate color change has been achieved in external process indicator immediately after removal from sterilizer then check internal process indicator before treatment. Refer to state regulations for any additional state requirements. Anesthetic cartridge and needle must be disposed of in a Sharps container. Refer to local and state recommendations for disposal of anesthetic cartridge. Dispose of topical in garbage. Single use only.

Evacuation Devices, Air/Water Syringe Tip, and Dental Unit

■INSTRUMENT # High-Volume (Velocity) Evacuator (HVE) Tip

Function ▶ To evacuate large volumes of fluid and debris from the oral cavity

Characteristics ▶
1 Stainless steel evacuator tip
2 Plastic evacuator tip—Disposable plastic

Straight or slightly angled at one or both ends
Also available in plastic that may be sterilized

Practice Notes ▶ Evacuator Tip attaches to high-velocity tubing on dental unit.
HVE Tip is used on most tray setups.

Sterilization Notes ▶ HVE Tip must be precleaned, either, placed in a sterilizing pouch with an internal process indicator, sealed, then sterilized OR wrapped with an internal process indicator inside and secured on the outside with process indicator tape, then sterilized. Verify appropriate color change has been achieved in external process indicator immediately after removal from sterilizer then check internal process indicator before treatment. Refer to state regulations for any additional state requirements. Disposable plastic HVE tip should be disposed of in the garbage.

Low-Volume (Velocity) Saliva Ejector Tip

Function ▶ To evacuate smaller volumes of fluid from the oral cavity

Characteristics ▶ Disposable plastic for single use only
Can be bent for placement under tongue and in other areas of mouth or can be used straight
Variety of styles

Practice Notes ▶ Attaches to low-velocity tubing on dental unit
Saliva Ejector Tip is used on most tray setups.

Sterilization Notes ▶ Disposable Saliva Ejector Tip should be disposed of in the garbage. Single use only. Refer to the Centers for Disease Control and Prevention (CDC) guidelines regarding possible backflow from low-volume saliva ejectors.

Isolite®—Illuminated Dental Isolation System

Functions ▶
To retract tongue and evacuate fluid from patient's mouth
To provide light to the working area of the mouth
To gently hold patient's mouth open during use
To serve as a barrier to the airway, protecting the patient from
inadvertent aspiration of dental material

Characteristics ▶
Isolite is attached to high-velocity evacuation port of the vacuum
system.
No special devices are required to operate system installed on
the dental unit.

Practice Notes ▶
Isolates two quadrants at once on the same side
Used for maxillary and mandibular procedures
Light settings for light-sensitive curing material

Sterilization Notes ▶
Please follow manufacturer's instructions for cleaning and sterilization. Applicable components should
be placed in sterilization pouch/bag and sealed or wrapped and secured with processing indicating tape,
then sterilized. An internal processing indicator should be included with each sterilization pouch and/or
wrap. When an internal processing indicator is not visible, then an external processing indicator should
be placed on the outside of the packaging. Indicators should be checked immediately upon removal
from sterilizer to verify the appropriate color change has been achieved. Refer to state regulations for
any additional state requirements. Disposable plastic should be disposed of in the garbage. Single use
only. Refer to manufacturer's recommendation and the CDC guidelines.

Low-Volume (Velocity) Mandibular Evacuator

Functions ►
To evacuate smaller volumes of fluid from the oral cavity
To use on mandibular arch
To retract tongue during evacuation

Characteristics ►
1 Blade for retraction of tongue is covered for patient comfort
2 Adjustable device to place under patient's chin to hold evacuator in place
Disposable plastic for single use only (may be referred to as a Linqua-fix)
Also available in metal, referred to as a Svedopter, must be sterilized

Practice Notes ►
Attaches to low-velocity tubing on dental unit
Disposable Low-Volume Mandibular Evacuator is used on sealant tray setups and on procedures for mandibular arch when operator is working without an assistant.
Disposable Low-Volume Mandibular Evacuator (pictured) should be disposed of in the garbage.

Sterilization Notes ►
Disposable Low-Volume Mandibular Evacuator should be disposed of in the garbage. Single use only. Svedopter (metal evacuator—not shown) must be precleaned, either, placed in a sterilizing pouch with an internal process indicator, sealed, then sterilized OR wrapped with an internal process indicator inside and secured on the outside with process indicator tape, then sterilized. Verify appropriate color change has been achieved in external process indicator immediately after removal from sterilizer then check internal process indicator before treatment. Refer to state regulations for any additional state requirements.

High-Volume (Velocity) Surgical Evacuation Tip

Function ▶ To evacuate fluid from oral cavity and surgical site

Characteristics ▶ Stainless steel, autoclavable plastic, disposable plastic:

  1 Stainless steel evacuation tip
  2 Plastic disposable tip

Narrowed tip accommodates surgical site.

Practice Notes ▶ Surgical evacuation tip attaches to high-velocity tubing on dental unit.

May require connecting tube for adaptation to surgical evacuation tip

Some stainless steel surgical tips narrow at insertion of tubing; additional tubing is necessary to connect to high-velocity tubing on dental unit.

Surgical Evacuation Tip is used on most surgical tray setups.

Sterilization Notes ▶ Surgical (Metal) Evacuation Tips must be precleaned, either, placed in a sterilizing pouch with an internal process indicator, sealed, then sterilized OR wrapped with an internal process indicator inside and secured on the outside with process indicator tape, then sterilized. Verify appropriate color change has been achieved in external process indicator immediately after removal from sterilizer then check internal process indicator before treatment. Refer to state regulations for any additional state requirements. Disposable Surgical Evacuation Tip should be disposed of in the garbage. Single use only.

Air/Water Syringe with Removable Tip

Function ▶ To rinse and dry specific teeth or entire oral cavity

Characteristics ▶ Air/water syringe is also referred to as a three-way syringe.
Characteristics of buttons on air/water syringe: left button expels water only; right button expels air only; pressing both buttons at the same time will result in a spray by combining air and water.
Types of tips:

1 Disposable plastic syringe tip for single use
2 Metal syringe tip
3 Seal-Tight tip seals water passage from getting into the air passage of the tip

Practice Notes ▶ Syringe Tip—Attaches to air/water syringe
Air/Water Syringe—Attaches to tubing on dental unit

Sterilization Notes ▶ Metal Air/Water Syringe Tip must be precleaned, either, placed in a sterilizing pouch with an internal process indicator, sealed, then sterilized OR wrapped with an internal process indicator inside and secured on the outside with process indicator tape, then sterilized. Verify appropriate color change has been achieved in external process indicator immediately after removal from sterilizer then check internal process indicator before treatment. Refer to state regulations for any additional state requirements. Disposable air/water syringe tip should be disposed of in the garbage. Single use only. Air/water syringe that tip is attached to must be disinfected according to manufacturer's recommendation.

73

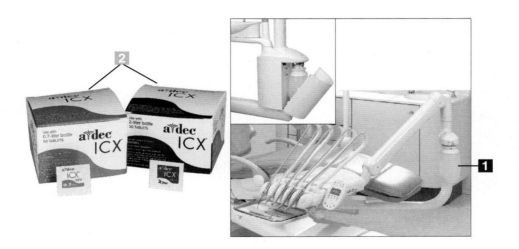

Self-Contained Water Unit and Waterline Treatment Tablets

Functions ► To assist in the quality of water entering the dental unit that supplies water to handpieces, air/water syringe, and cuspidor cupfill

To assist when there is a possibility of contamination to the water supply to the dental unit

Characteristics ► Water system may be mounted in different areas of the dental unit.

Different size bottles are available.

Example: 7 L or 2 L

1 Self-contained water bottle attached to dental unit

2 Tablets—Place tablets in each water bottle every time bottle is filled.

Reduces accumulation of contaminants

Reduces accumulation of order and foul-tasting bacteria

Practice Notes ► Follow manufacturer's recommendations for periodic shock treatment of water lines using special tablets; safety precautions while using tablets and filling bottles.

Sterilization Notes ► CDC recommends monitoring dental unit water regularly. Example weekly testing of water either in office or commercial monitoring system (Guidelines for Infection Control in Dental Health Care Setting, 2003).

■INSTRUMENT Dental Delivery System

Function ▶ To deliver dental care to patients

Characteristics ▶
1. Ergonomically structured chair for patient, operator, and assistant
2. Chair adjustment device for height and reclining patient
3. Light with adjustable intensity - LED light with curing option for composite restorations
4. Tubing for high and slow speed handpieces, air/water syringe, low- and high-velocity vacuum systems
5. Rheostat for running handpieces with water toggle switch option
6. Tray for placing instrument setups
7. Computer screen available for patient information and digital images

Practice Notes ▶ Many different designs of dental delivery systems available
Air/water syringes available on one or both sides of operator or assistant's side
Evacuation tubing on assistant's side of patient chair
Tubing for handpieces available on operator or assistant's side of patient chair

Sterilization Notes ▶ Refer to manufacturing and CDC guidelines on purging dental lines (tubing), disinfecting chair, tubing, and dental unit.

∎INSTRUMENT Dental Assistant Delivery System

Function ▸ To deliver dental care to patients as a chairside assistant

Characteristics ▸
1. Saliva ejector attached to the low-volume evacuation system tubing
2. Air/water syringe and tip attached to the tubing
3. High-volume evacuator tip attached to the tubing
4. Light curing device attached to the unit with protective shield
5. Bracket table for instrument setups
6. Chair adjustment device for height and reclining dental chair

Practice Notes ▸ Many different designs of dental delivery systems are available. Dental assistant delivery system is used to deliver dental care to patients.

Sterilization Notes ▸ Refer to manufacturing and CDC guidelines on purging dental lines (tubing), tubing, and disinfecting delivery system.

▪INSTRUMENT Dental Stools

Function ▶ To use providing treatment to a patient

Characteristics ▶
1. Operator chair—adjustable back support is movable forward and backward
2. Operator and Assistant chair—adjustable seat height
3. Adjustable torso support
4. Assistant chair—adjustable foot ring under seat for feet support

Practice Notes ▶ Operator chair—Feet recommended to be placed flat on floor for ergonomically correct position

Assistant chair—Feet recommended to be place on ring, bar underneath rib cage; while seated in the chair the assistant should be 4 to 6 inches above operator for ergonomically correct position.

Sterilization Notes ▶ Chairs must be disinfected (including the height adjustment lever) after each patient; refer to manufacturer's recommendation for disinfection of chairs.

Dental Handpieces

High-Speed Handpiece

Functions ► To use with bur to cut tooth structure, to cut bone, to remove decay, and to modify or remove restorations
Example: Cavity preparation for restoration or crown
To use with bur for adjusting crowns and bridges for final fit

Characteristics ► Handpiece is run by air pressure at a maximum speed of 450,000 rotations per minute (rpm).
On high-speed handpiece, bur generates extreme amount of heat.
Instrument sprays water/air or air on bur for cooling purposes to prevent damage to pulp.
Different styles of securing bur are available:

1 Power lever chuck 2 Push-button chuck
3 Conventional chuck—Need to secure bur and loosen bur in handpiece with wrench

Practice Notes ► Handpiece attaches to tubing on dental unit.

Sterilization Notes ► Most High-Speed Handpiece must be lubricated and precleaned according to the manufacturer's recommendation. Then, either, placed in a sterilizing pouch with an internal process indicator, sealed, then sterilized OR wrapped with an internal process indicator inside and secured on the outside with process indicator tape, then sterilized. Verify appropriate color change has been achieved in external process indicator immediately after removal from sterilizer then check internal process indicator before treatment. Refer to state regulations for any additional state requirements.

Fiberoptic High-Speed Handpiece

Functions ▶ To illuminate tooth during preparation for restoration
To provide light intraorally during use of handpiece
To use with bur to cut tooth structure, to cut bone, to
remove decay, and to modify or remove restorations
Example: Cavity preparation for restoration or crown
To use with bur for adjusting crowns and bridges for
final fit

Characteristics ▶ **1** Light(s) at head of handpiece

Lights up working area while handpiece rotates
Same characteristics as high-speed handpiece

Practice Notes ▶ Handpiece attaches to tubing on dental unit.
Tubing has special adaptor for light availability.

Sterilization Notes ▶ Most fiberoptic High-Speed Handpiece must be lubricated and precleaned according to the
manufacturer's recommendation. Then, must be either, placed in a sterilizing pouch with
an internal process indicator, sealed, then sterilized OR wrapped with an internal process
indicator inside and secured on the outside with process indicator tape, then sterilized. Verify
appropriate color change has been achieved in external process indicator immediately after
removal from sterilizer then check internal process indicator before treatment.
Refer to state regulations for any additional state requirements.

Forward

Reverse

Slow-Speed Motor with Straight Handpiece Attachment

Functions ▶ To use with slow-speed attachments
To use straight attachment with long-shank straight bur

Characteristics ▶ **1** Slow-speed motor
2 Straight handpiece attachment (with bur attached)

Maximum speed of 30,000 rpm; used as adjunct to high-speed handpiece
Straight attachment—Used outside oral cavity, usually in a laboratory setting
Contra-angle or prophy angle attachments—Designed for intraoral use
Handpiece must be engaged in either forward or reverse.

Practice Notes ▶ Slow-Speed Motor attaches to tubing on dental unit.

Sterilization Notes ▶ Slow-Speed Motor with Straight Handpiece Attachment must be lubricated and precleaned according to the manufacturer's recommendation. Then, must be either, placed in a sterilizing pouch with an internal process indicator, sealed, then sterilized OR wrapped with an internal process indicator inside and secured on the outside with process indicator tape, then sterilized. Verify appropriate color change has been achieved in external process indicator immediately after removal from sterilizer then check internal process indicator before treatment. Refer to state regulations for any additional state requirements.

Slow-Speed Motor with Contra-Angle Handpiece Attachment

Functions ▶ To use with burs for intraoral and extraoral procedures to remove decay, polish amalgam restorations, refine cavity preparation, adjust provisional and permanent crowns and bridges, adjust occlusal restorations, adjust partials and dentures, and to provide prophylaxis treatment

Characteristics ▶
1 Contra-angle attachment
2 Slow-speed motor
3 Push-button device to secure bur—Using friction grip bur

4 Latch-type attachment—Using latch-type bur
Top: latch open; *Bottom:* latch closed

Contra-angle attaches to straight handpiece or to Slow-Speed Motor.
Types of Contra-Angle Attachments:
- Latch type—Latch-type bur, prophylaxis polishing cup or brush. Bur is secured by swivel of latch-type device in back of handpiece.
- Friction grip—Friction grip bur. Bur is secured by pushing back of handpiece.

Practice Notes ▶ Slow-Speed Motor attaches to tubing on dental unit.
Sterilization Notes ▶ Slow-Speed Motor with Contra-Angle Handpiece Attachment must be lubricated and precleaned according to the manufacturer's recommendation. Then, must be either, placed in a sterilizing pouch with an internal process indicator, sealed, then sterilized OR wrapped with an internal process indicator inside and secured on the outside with process indicator tape, then sterilized. Verify appropriate color change has been achieved in external process indicator immediately after removal from sterilizer then check internal process indicator before treatment. Refer to state regulations for any additional state requirements.

Prophy Slow-Speed Handpiece/Motor* with Disposable Prophy Angle Attachment

Function ▶ To polish teeth with prophylaxis/prophy cup or brush attachment

Characteristics ▶

1 Disposable prophy angle attachment (with rubber polishing cup)

2 Prophy Slow-Speed Handpiece/Motor

Prophy angle attaches to handpiece/motor.

Ergonomic shape for natural hand positioning

Lightweight design to reduce hand and wrist fatigue

Practice Notes ▶ Prophy Slow-Speed Handpiece/Motor attaches to tubing on dental unit.

Sterilization Notes ▶ Prophy Slow-Speed Handpiece/Motor must be lubricated and precleaned according to the manufacturer's recommendation. Then, must be either, placed in a sterilizing pouch with an internal process indicator, sealed, then sterilized OR wrapped with an internal process indicator inside and secured on the outside with process indicator tape, then sterilized. Verify appropriate color change has been achieved in external process indicator immediately after removal from sterilizer then check internal process indicator before treatment. Refer to state regulations for any additional state requirements.

* Referred to as RDH (Registered Dental Hygiene) Prophy Angle.

Rechargeable Prophy Slow-Speed Handpiece/ Motor- RDH Freedom™

Function ▶ To polish teeth for prophylaxis with prophy cup and/or brush

Characteristics ▶ **1** Foot Pedal-Wireless-Cordless rechargeable
To operate Foot Pedal and control speed of handpiece
RDH Freedom™ Cordless Rechargable Prophy Handpiece.
Parts:
2 Sheath—Handpiece Attachment
3 Motor
4 Cradle to hold the handpiece
Types of Prophy Angle Attachments:
Disposable prophy cup—For polishing all surfaces of teeth
Disposable prophy brush—For polishing occlusal surfaces and deep grooves on lingual surfaces of anterior teeth

Practice Notes ▶ Rechargeable handpiece is used mostly on prophylaxis and sealant tray setups.

Sterilization Notes ▶ Motor should have a barrier otherwise follow manufacture's recommendation for lubricating, precleaning, and sterilization. Sheath must be either, placed in a sterilizing pouch with an internal process indicator, sealed, then sterilized OR wrapped with an internal process indicator inside and secured on the outside with process indicator tape, then sterilized. Verify appropriate color change has been achieved in external process indicator immediately after removal from sterilizer then check internal process indicator before treatment. Disposable prophy angle attachments -rubber polishing cup or brush- must be disposed of in garbage. Single use only. Cradle should have a barrier or otherwise disinfect according to manufacturer's recommendation.

Disposable Prophy Angle Attachments for Slow-Speed Handpiece/Motor

Function ▶ To polish teeth for prophylaxis

Characteristics ▶ Attaches to straight or prophy slow-speed handpiece/motor

Types:

1 Disposable prophy angle attachment with prophy cup. Prophy cup—Variety of flexibility and designs available for polishing all surfaces of teeth.

2 Disposable prophy angle attachment with tapered brush—For polishing occlusal surfaces and deep grooves on lingual surfaces of anterior teeth.

Practice Note ▶ Disposable Prophy Angle Attachments are used mostly on prophylaxis and sealant tray setups.

Sterilization Notes ▶ Disposable Prophy Angle Attachments (rubber polishing cup or brush) must be disposed of in garbage. Single use only.

Prophy Angle Slow-Speed Handpiece/Motor*

Function ▶ To polish teeth for prophylaxis

Characteristics ▶ Prophy angle slow-speed handpiece/motor is one piece.
Disposable screw-type prophy cup or brush attaches to prophy angle slow-speed handpiece/motor.
Lightweight design to reduce hand and wrist fatigue
Ergonomic shape for natural hand positioning
Attachments:

1 Flat-end brush
2 Tapered-end brush
3 Prophy cup—Variety of flexibility and designs available

Practice Note ▶ Prophy Angle Slow-Speed Handpiece/Motor attaches to tubing on dental unit.

Sterilization Notes ▶ Prophy Angle Slow-Speed Handpiece/Motor must be lubricated and precleaned according to the manufacturer's recommendation. Then, must be either, placed in a sterilizing pouch with an internal process indicator, sealed, then sterilized OR wrapped with an internal process indicator inside and secured on the outside with process indicator tape, then sterilized. Verify appropriate color change has been achieved in external process indicator immediately after removal from sterilizer then check internal process indicator before treatment. Refer to state regulations for any additional state requirements. Disposable prophy polishing cup or brush must be disposed of in garbage. Single use only.

*Referred to as an RDH (Registered Dental Hygienist) prophy handpiece.

Electric Handpiece Unit and Handpiece Attachments

Functions ▶ To use with bur for intraoral cavity preparation

To use with endodontic nickel-titanium rotary instruments

To use with bur for trimming of provisional crowns

To use with bur for adjusting permanent restorations, crowns, and bridges

Characteristics ▶
1 Electric Handpiece Unit

2 Electric Handpiece Attachments

3 Electric Handpiece Motor

Speed of handpiece can be set to specific rpms.

Practice Notes ▶ Handpiece attaches to tubing on electric handpiece unit.

Electric Handpiece is used with restorative, endodontic, and surgical tray setups.

Sterilization Notes ▶ Electric Handpiece Motor must be lubricated and precleaned according to the manufacturer's recommendation. Then, Motor and Attachments must either, placed in a sterilizing pouch with an internal process indicator, sealed, then sterilized OR wrapped with an internal process indicator inside and secured on the outside with process indicator tape, then sterilized. Verify appropriate color change has been achieved in external process indicator immediately after removal from sterilizer then check internal process indicator before treatment. Refer to state regulations for any additional state requirements. Barriers should be used on the unit, or the manufacturer's recommendation should be followed for disinfecting the unit.

▪INSTRUMENT Surgical Electrical Handpiece Unit and Handpiece Attachments

Functions ▶
1. To use with depth drills for implants
2. To use with sterile water for cooling drilling system

Characteristics ▶ Straight and contra-angled (pictured) handpiece attachments available
Maximum speed of 40,000 rpm
Lower speed (e.g., 10–50 rpm) used for implant
Fiberoptic light available for these handpieces

Practice Note ▶ Surgical Electrical Handpiece Unit and Handpiece Attachments are used with surgical tray setups.

Sterilization Notes ▶ Surgical Electrical Handpiece Motor must be lubricated and precleaned according to the manufacturer's recommendation. Then, Motor and Attachments must either, placed in a sterilizing pouch with an internal process indicator, sealed, then sterilized OR wrapped with an internal process indicator inside and secured on the outside with process indicator tape, then sterilized. Verify appropriate color change has been achieved in external process indicator immediately after removal from sterilizer then check internal process indicator before treatment. Barriers should be used on the unit, or the manufacturer's recommendation should be followed for disinfecting the unit. Sterile water single use only.

■INSTRUMENT Air Abrasion Unit and Handpiece Attachment

Functions ▶ To use for class I through class VI cavity preparation
To use for preparation of occlusal surface for sealants

Characteristics ▶ Handpiece attachment uses high pressure of alpha-alumina particles through small device that removes decay or prepares pit and fissures for sealants or restoration.
Minimal use of anesthesia is required.

Practice Note ▶ Air Abrasion Unit and Handpiece Attachment are used with class I through class VI restorative tray setups and with sealant tray setups.

Sterilization Notes ▶ Air Abrasion Handpiece Attachments must be lubricated and precleaned according to the manufacturer's recommendation. Then, either, placed in a sterilizing pouch with an internal process indicator, sealed, then sterilized OR wrapped with an internal process indicator inside and secured on the outside with process indicator tape, then sterilized. Verify appropriate color change has been achieved in external process indicator immediately after removal from sterilizer then check internal process indicator before treatment. Refer to state regulations for any additional state requirements. Barriers should be used on the unit, or the manufacturer's recommendation should be followed for disinfecting the unit.

■INSTRUMENT Air Polisher

Function ▶ To polish teeth by directing a high-pressure jet of pressurized air, water and mild polishing agent of sodium bicarbonate

Characteristics ▶

1. Combination of slurry of water and powder cleans or debrides the tooth surface utilizing the Air Polisher Tip

2. Foot Pedal that controls the Air Polisher

Air Polisher has a self-contained water reservoir.
Air Polisher is connected to the dental unit water supply tubing.

Practice Note ▶ Air Polisher used in place of polishing teeth with prophy paste, prophy cup, and brush.

Sterilization Notes ▶ Air Polisher Unit Attachment tips must be precleaned, either, placed in a sterilizing pouch with an internal process indicator, sealed, then sterilized OR wrapped with an internal process indicator inside and secured on the outside with process indicator tape, then sterilized. Verify appropriate color change has been achieved in external process indicator immediately after removal from sterilizer then check internal process indicator before treatment. Refer to state regulations for any additional state requirements. Barriers should be used on the unit, and attachments or the manufacturer's recommendation should be followed for disinfecting the unit and attachments.

Handpiece Maintenance System

Function ▸ To flush internal air/water coolant lines on high- and slow-speed handpieces
To remove debris within handpiece and prevent buildup
To lubricate handpiece

Characteristics ▸
1 Cover encloses system
2 Under cover connection for handpieces—Lift cover to access
3 Start button
4 Filter system

Universal adaptor for many styles of handpieces
Cleans and lubricates before bagging to sterilized
Keeps aerosols contained and filters exhaust and air from unit

Practice Note ▸ To use, connect the instrument and close the cover and then push the start button for 2 seconds to begin automated delivery of service oil and cleaning liquid; cycle is complete in 35 seconds. Also refer to the instruction manual of the handpiece as different handpieces have to be lubricated different ways and at different times.

Sterilization Notes ▸ Refer to the manufacturer's recommendations for cleaning and disinfecting.

Laser Handpiece Unit and Laser Handpiece Attachment

Function ▶ To cut, vaporize, or cauterize soft tissue
Examples:

  To remove lesions or tumors
  To reduce excess tissue
  To control bleeding

Characteristics ▶ Works by means of a highly concentrated light source
SIROLaser (pictured) operates at a wavelength of 980 nanometers and has a power output varying from 0.5 to 7 watts.

Practice Notes ▶ Laser Handpiece Unit and Laser Handpiece Attachment are used with specialty procedures.
Examples: Prosthodontics and Oral Surgery

Sterilization Notes ▶ Laser Handpiece must be lubricated and prcleaned according to the manufacturer's recommendation. Then, either, placed in a sterilizing pouch with an internal process indicator, sealed, then sterilized OR wrapped with an internal process indicator inside and secured on the outside with process indicator tape, then sterilized. Verify appropriate color change has been achieved in external process indicator immediately after removal from sterilizer then check internal process indicator before treatment. Refer to state regulations for any additional state requirements. Barriers should be used on the unit, or the manufacturer's recommendation should be followed for disinfecting the unit.

Dental Unit

Functions ▶

1 To provide a delivery system for handpieces and air/water syringe
2 To provide delivery system for air/water syringe
3 To provide intraoral camera
4 To provide a device for moving dental chair up, down, forward, and backward

Characteristics ▶ Delivery systems provide at least two tubings—one for high-speed handpieces and one for slow-speed handpiece. Above illustrates two tubing unit.
Special mechanism required for fiberoptic handpiece

Practice Notes ▶ Different designs of dental delivery systems available in front, rear or side delivery
Air/water syringes available on one or both sides of operator or assistant's side

Barriers should be used on tubing, or the manufacturer's recommendation should be followed for disinfecting unit and tubing. All handpiece attachments and handpieces must be lubricated and precleaned according to the manufacturer's recommendation. Then, either, placed in a sterilizing pouch with an internal process indicator, sealed, then sterilized OR wrapped with an internal process indicator inside and secured on the outside with process indicator tape, then sterilized. Verify appropriate color change has been achieved in external process indicator immediately after removal from sterilizer then check internal process indicator before treatment. Refer to state regulations for any additional state requirements.

Burs and Rotary Attachments for Handpieces

Bur

Function ▶ To be used in a high- or low-speed handpiece

Characteristics ▶ Parts:

1 Head: Part of bur that cuts, polishes, or finishes

- Available in a variety of shapes and sizes

2 Neck: Part of bur that tapers to connect shank to head

3 Shank: Part of bur that is inserted into the handpiece

- Length and style of shank vary depending on handpiece used.
- Bur with straight, long shank fits into straight slow-speed handpiece.
- Bur with latch-type shank fits into contra-angle slow-speed handpiece (friction grip bur shown).
- Friction grip bur fits into high-speed handpiece; chuck, lever, or push button tightens bur into the handpiece.
- Bur with long shank used for surgical procedures

Sterilization Notes ▶ Burs must be precleaned, either, placed in a sterilizing pouch with an internal process indicator, sealed, then sterilized OR wrapped with an internal process indicator inside and secured on the outside with process indicator tape, then sterilized. Verify appropriate color change has been achieved in external process indicator immediately after removal from sterilizer then check internal process indicator before treatment. Refer to state regulations for any additional state requirements. Or, the used bur must be disposed of in a sharps container.

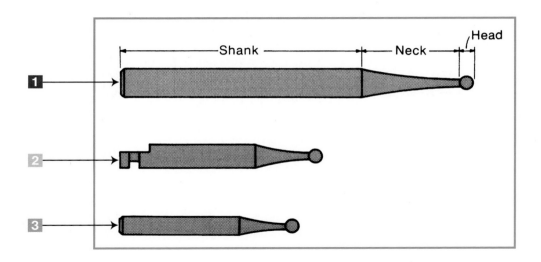

| ▪INSTRUMENT | # Bur Shanks |

Function ▶ To fit shank part of bur into handpiece

Characteristics ▶ Fit a variety of shanks into different styles of handpieces

Working or cutting end of the bur could be the same style or size, but shank could be different according to handpiece used

Examples:

1 No. 2 round bur in straight shank
2 No. 2 round bur in latch shank
3 No. 2 round bur in friction grip shank

Long shank used for surgical procedures

Sterilization Notes ▶ Burs must be precleaned, either, placed in a sterilizing pouch with an internal process indicator, sealed, then sterilized OR wrapped with an internal process indicator inside and secured on the outside with process indicator tape, then sterilized. Verify appropriate color change has been achieved in external process indicator immediately after removal from sterilizer then check internal process indicator before treatment. Refer to state regulations for any additional state requirements. Or, the used bur must be disposed of in a sharps container.

Round Bur

Functions ▶ To remove caries from tooth structure
To open tooth for endodontic treatment
To create retention in cavity preparation
To use for many procedures on a tooth

Characteristics ▶ Range of sizes
Commonly used sizes: No. 1/4 to No. 10

Practice Notes ▶ Bur is inserted and secured in a handpiece.
Type of handpiece determines type of shank used.

Sterilization Notes ▶ A Round Bur must be precleaned, either, placed in a sterilizing
pouch with an internal process indicator, sealed, then sterilized OR
wrapped with an internal process indicator inside and secured on the
outside with process indicator tape, then sterilized. Verify appropriate color change has been
achieved in external process indicator immediately after removal from sterilizer then check
internal process indicator before treatment. Refer to state regulations for any additional state
requirements. Or, the used bur must be disposed of in a sharps container.

Pear-Shaped Bur

Functions ▶ To open tooth for a restoration
To remove caries

Characteristics ▶ Frequently used in preparation of composite restorations
Range of sizes
Commonly used sizes: No. 330 to No. 333
Bur head available in long
Example: No. 333L

Practice Notes ▶ Bur is inserted and secured in a handpiece.
Type of handpiece determines type of shank used.

Sterilization Notes ▶ Pear-Shaped Bur must be precleaned, either, placed in a sterilizing pouch with an internal process indicator, sealed, then sterilized OR wrapped with an internal process indicator inside and secured on the outside with process indicator tape, then sterilized. Verify appropriate color change has been achieved in external process indicator immediately after removal from sterilizer then check internal process indicator before treatment. Refer to state regulations for any additional state requirements. Or, the used bur must be disposed of in a sharps container.

Inverted Cone Bur

Functions ▶ To remove caries
To establish retention in tooth for cavity preparation

Characteristics ▶ Range of sizes
Commonly used sizes: No. 33½, No. 34, No. 37, No. 39

Practice Notes ▶ Bur is inserted and secured in a handpiece.
Type of handpiece determines type of shank used.

Sterilization Notes ▶ Inverted Cone Bur must be precleaned, either, placed
in a sterilizing pouch with an internal process indicator,
sealed, then sterilized OR wrapped with an internal process
indicator inside and secured on the outside with process
indicator tape, then sterilized. Verify appropriate color
change has been achieved in external process indicator
immediately after removal from sterilizer then check internal process indicator before
treatment. Refer to state regulations for any additional state requirements. Or, the used bur
must be disposed of in a sharps container.

∎INSTRUMENT Straight Fissure Bur—Plain Cut

Functions ▶
To cut cavity preparation
To form inner walls of cavity preparation
To create retention grooves in walls of cavity preparation

Characteristics ▶
Cutting part of bur—Has parallel sides
Range of sizes—Commonly used: No. 56, No. 57, No. 58
May have short or long (L) shank for adaptation to a variety
of cavity preparations
Examples of short and long shank friction grip burs: No. 56S,
No. 56L

Practice Notes ▶
Bur is inserted and secured in a handpiece.
Type of handpiece determines type of shank used.

Sterilization Notes ▶
Straight Fissure Bur—Plain Cut must be precleaned, either, placed in a sterilizing pouch
with an internal process indicator, sealed, then sterilized OR wrapped with an internal
process indicator inside and secured on the outside with process indicator tape, then
sterilized. Verify appropriate color change has been achieved in external process indicator
immediately after removal from sterilizer then check internal process indicator before
treatment. Refer to state regulations for any additional state requirements. Or, the used bur
must be disposed of in a sharps container.

Tapered Fissure Bur—Plain Cut

Functions ▶ To cut cavity preparation
To form angles in walls of cavity preparation
To place retention grooves in walls of cavity preparation

Characteristics ▶ Cutting part of bur—Has tapered sides
Range of sizes—Commonly used: No. 168, No. 169, No. 170, No. 171
May have short (S) or long (L) shank for adaptation to a variety of
cavity preparations
Examples of short and long shank friction grip burs: No. 168S, No.
171L

Practice Notes ▶ Bur is inserted and secured in a handpiece.
Type of handpiece determines type of shank used.

Sterilization Notes ▶ Tapered Fissure Bur—Plain Cut must be precleaned, either, placed
in a sterilizing pouch with an internal process indicator, sealed, then sterilized OR wrapped
with an internal process indicator inside and secured on the outside with process indicator
tape, then sterilized. Verify appropriate color change has been achieved in external process
indicator immediately after removal from sterilizer then check internal process indicator
before treatment. Refer to state regulations for any additional state requirements. Refer to
state regulations for any additional state requirements. Or, used bur must be disposed of in a
sharps container.

Straight Fissure Bur—Crosscut

Functions ▶ To cut cavity preparation
To form walls of cavity preparation
To create retention grooves in walls of cavity preparation

Characteristics ▶ Cutting part of bur—Has parallel sides with horizontal cutting
edges
Range of sizes—Commonly used: No. 556, No. 557, No. 558
May have long (L) shank for adaptation to a variety of cavity
preparations
Example of long shank friction grip bur: No. 556L

Practice Notes ▶ Bur is inserted and secured in a handpiece.
Type of handpiece determines type of shank used.

Sterilization Notes ▶ Straight Fissure Bur—Crosscut must be precleaned, either, placed in a sterilizing pouch with
an internal process indicator, sealed, then sterilized OR wrapped with an internal process
indicator inside and secured on the outside with process indicator tape, then sterilized.
Verify appropriate color change has been achieved in external process indicator immediately
after removal from sterilizer then check internal process indicator before treatment. Refer to
state regulations for any additional state requirements. Or, the used bur must be disposed of
in a sharps container.

Tapered Fissure Bur—Crosscut

Functions ▶
To cut cavity preparation
To form angles in walls of cavity preparation
To create retention grooves in walls of cavity preparation

Characteristics ▶
Cutting part of bur—Has tapered sides with horizontal cutting edges
Range of sizes—Commonly used: No. 699, No. 700, No. 701, No. 702, No. 703
May have long (L) shank for adaptation to a variety of cavity preparations
Example of long shank friction grip bur: No. 701L

Practice Notes ▶
Bur is inserted and secured in a handpiece.
Type of handpiece determines type of shank used.

Sterilization Notes ▶
Tapered Fissure Bur—Crosscut must be precleaned, either, placed in a sterilizing pouch with an internal process indicator, sealed, then sterilized OR wrapped with an internal process indicator inside and secured on the outside with process indicator tape, then sterilized. Verify appropriate color change has been achieved in external process indicator immediately after removal from sterilizer then check internal process indicator before treatment. Refer to state regulations for any additional state requirements. Or, the used bur must be disposed of in a sharps container.

Finishing Bur

Functions ▶ To finish composite restoration
To finish restoration by restoring anatomy in tooth
To equilibrate or adjust occlusion

Characteristic ▶ Variety of shapes and sizes
Finishing bur differs from the cutting burs as the working end or cutting end has an increased number of blades or flutes. An increased amount of blades will determine the greater amount of polishing capabilities.

Practice Notes ▶ Bur is inserted and secured in a handpiece.
Type of handpiece determines type of shank used.

Sterilization Notes ▶ Finishing Bur must be precleaned, either, placed in a
sterilizing pouch with an internal process indicator, sealed, then sterilized OR wrapped with an internal process indicator inside and secured on the outside with process indicator tape, then sterilized. Verify appropriate color change has been achieved in external process indicator immediately after removal from sterilizer then check internal process indicator before treatment. Refer to state regulations for any additional state requirements. Or, the used bur must be disposed of in a sharps container.

Diamond Bur—Flat-End Taper

Function ▶ To reduce a tooth for crown preparation when a square shoulder is needed

Characteristics ▶ Range of grits—Superfine to coarse; grit designated by color band on shank of diamond bur or by letter after name of diamond bur
Superfine diamond burs—Used for finishing restorations
Variety of shapes and sizes

Practice Notes ▶ Bur is inserted and secured in a handpiece.
Type of handpiece determines type of shank used.

Sterilization Notes ▶ Diamond Bur—Flat-End Taper must be precleaned, either, placed in a sterilizing pouch with an internal process indicator, sealed, then sterilized OR wrapped with an internal process indicator inside and secured on the outside with process indicator tape, then sterilized. Verify appropriate color change has been achieved in external process indicator immediately after removal from sterilizer then check internal process indicator before treatment. Refer to state regulations for any additional state requirements. Or, the used diamond bur must be disposed of in a sharps container.

Diamond Bur—Flat-End Cylinder

Function ▶ To reduce a tooth for crown preparation when parallel walls and flat floors are needed

Characteristics ▶ Range of grits—Superfine to coarse; grit designated by color band on shank of diamond bur or by letter after name of diamond bur
Superfine diamond burs—Used for finishing restorations
Variety of shapes and sizes

Practice Notes ▶ Bur is inserted and secured in a handpiece.
Type of handpiece determines type of shank used.

Sterilization Notes ▶ Diamond Bur—Flat-End Cylinder must be precleaned, either, placed in a sterilizing pouch with an internal process indicator, sealed, then sterilized OR wrapped with an internal process indicator inside and secured on the outside with process indicator tape, then sterilized. Verify appropriate color change has been achieved in external process indicator immediately after removal from sterilizer then check internal process indicator before treatment. Refer to state regulations for any additional state requirements. Or, the used bur must be disposed of in a sharps container.

Diamond Bur—Flame

Function ▶ To reduce a tooth for crown preparation for subgingival margins

Characteristics ▶ Range of grits—Superfine to coarse; grit designated by color band on shank of diamond bur or by letter after name of diamond bur
Superfine diamond burs—Used for finishing restorations
Variety of shapes and sizes

Practice Notes ▶ Bur is inserted and secured in a handpiece.
Type of handpiece determines type of shank used.

Sterilization Notes ▶ Diamond Bur—Flame must be precleaned, either, placed in a sterilizing pouch with an internal process indicator, sealed, then sterilized OR wrapped with an internal process indicator inside and secured on the outside with process indicator tape, then sterilized. Verify appropriate color change has been achieved in external process indicator immediately after removal from sterilizer then check internal process indicator before treatment. Refer to state regulations for any additional state requirements. Or, the used bur must be disposed of in a sharps container.

Diamond Bur—Wheel

Function ▶ To reduce a tooth for crown preparation on lingual aspect of anterior teeth and to reduce bulk of incisal edges

Characteristics ▶ Range of grits—Superfine to coarse; grit designated by color band on shank of diamond bur or by letter after name of diamond bur
Superfine diamond burs—Used for finishing restorations
Variety of shapes and sizes

Practice Notes ▶ Bur is inserted and secured in a handpiece.
Type of handpiece determines type of shank used.

Sterilization Notes ▶ Diamond Bur—Wheel must be precleaned, either, placed in a sterilizing pouch with an internal process indicator, sealed, then sterilized OR wrapped with an internal process indicator inside and secured on the outside with process indicator tape, then sterilized. Verify appropriate color change has been achieved in external process indicator immediately after removal from sterilizer then check internal process indicator before treatment. Refer to state regulations for any additional state requirements. Or, the used bur must be disposed of in a sharps container.

Mandrel—Snap On

Function ▶ To attach discs to mandrel for finishing and polishing inside or outside oral cavity (mandrel is inserted into handpiece)

Characteristics ▶ Shank types:

1 Long shank—For straight slow-speed handpiece
2 Short latch-type shank—For contra-angle slow-speed handpiece
3 Friction grip shank—For high-speed handpiece

Plastic disposable Snap on Mandrels available

Practice Notes ▶ Mandrel is inserted and secured in a handpiece.
Type of handpiece determines type of shank used.

Sterilization Notes ▶ Mandrel—Snap On must be precleaned, either, placed in a sterilizing pouch with an internal process indicator, sealed, then sterilized OR wrapped with an internal process indicator inside and secured on the outside with process indicator tape, then sterilized. Verify appropriate color change has been achieved in external process indicator immediately after removal from sterilizer then check internal process indicator before treatment. Refer to state regulations for any additional state requirements. Disposable snap-on mandrels should be disposed of in the garbage. Single use only.

Mandrel—Screw On

Function ▶ To attach discs to mandrel for finishing and polishing inside or outside oral cavity (mandrel is inserted into handpiece)

Characteristics ▶ Shank types:

1 Long shank—For straight slow-speed handpiece
2 Short latch-type shank—For contra-angle or right-angle slow-speed handpiece
3 Friction grip shank—For high-speed handpiece

Practice Notes ▶ Mandrel is inserted and secured in a handpiece.
Type of handpiece determines type of shank used.

Sterilization Notes ▶ Mandrel—Screw On must be precleaned, either, placed in a sterilizing pouch with an internal process indicator, sealed, then sterilized OR wrapped with an internal process indicator inside and secured on the outside with process indicator tape, then sterilized. Verify appropriate color change has been achieved in external process indicator immediately after removal from sterilizer then check internal process indicator before treatment. Refer to state regulations for any additional state requirements.

Sandpaper Disc with Screw-Type and Snap-On Mandrel

Functions ▶ To contour restorations
To polish restorative material (extra fine grit)

Characteristics ▶ Range of grits (coarse to extra fine)
Darker color of disc denotes more abrasiveness
Two types:

1 Screw on
2 Snap on (metal center)

Sandpaper Disc organizer has a range of sizes and grits.

Practice Notes ▶ Sandpaper Disc is attached to either a snap-on mandrel or a
screw-on mandrel, depending on the type of Sandpaper Disc
being used.

Sterilization Notes ▶ Disposable Sandpaper Discs should be disposed of in the
garbage. Mandrel must be precleaned, either, placed in a
sterilizing pouch with an internal process indicator, sealed, then sterilized OR wrapped
with an internal process indicator inside and secured on the outside with process indicator
tape, then sterilized. Verify appropriate color change has been achieved in external process
indicator immediately after removal from sterilizer then check internal process indicator
before treatment. Refer to state regulations for any additional state requirements.

1

2

Composite Disc

Functions ▶ To contour restorations
To polish or smooth restorative material (extra fine grit)

Characteristics ▶ Made from synthetic material to accommodate composite restorations
Range of grits (coarse to extra fine)
Darker color of disc denotes more abrasiveness
Variety of sizes
Two types available:

1 Snap on composite disc
2 Composite disc with disposable mandrel

Practice Notes ▶ Composite Disc is attached to either a snap-on mandrel or a screw-on mandrel, depending on the type of Composite Disc being used.

Sterilization Notes ▶ Disposable Composite Discs and disposable mandrel should be disposed of in the garbage. Single use only. Metal mandrel must be precleaned, either, placed in a sterilizing pouch with an internal process indicator, sealed, then sterilized OR wrapped with an internal process indicator inside and secured on the outside with process indicator tape, then sterilized. Verify appropriate color change has been achieved in external process indicator immediately after removal from sterilizer then check internal process indicator before treatment. Refer to state regulations for any additional state requirements.

■INSTRUMENT Rubber Points

Function ▶ To polish restorations, amalgam, composite, and gold

Characteristics ▶ Types of polishing grits:
Brown points (brownies)—Abrasive
Green points (greenies)—Less abrasive than brownies
White points—Polishing point
Variety of shanks available for all types of rubber points:

1 Friction grip
2 Latch type

Practice Notes ▶ Rubber Point is inserted and secured in a handpiece.
Type of handpiece determines type of shank used.

Sterilization Notes ▶ Rubber Point must be precleaned, either, placed in a sterilizing pouch with an internal process indicator, sealed, then sterilized OR wrapped with an internal process indicator inside and secured on the outside with process indicator tape, then sterilized. Verify appropriate color change has been achieved in external process indicator immediately after removal from sterilizer then check internal process indicator before treatment. Refer to state regulations for any additional state requirements.

Laboratory Bur—Acrylic Bur

Function ▶ To cut models or trim acrylic in laboratory

Characteristics ▶ Long shank—For attachment to straight handpiece
Variety of sizes and shapes

Practice Notes ▶ Laboratory Bur is inserted and secured in a slow-speed handpiece with a straight attachment.

Sterilization Notes ▶ Laboratory Bur—Acrylic Bur, when used on any patient's appliances must be precleaned, either, placed in a sterilizing pouch with an internal process indicator, sealed, then sterilized OR wrapped with an internal process indicator inside and secured on the outside with process indicator tape, then sterilized. Verify appropriate color change has been achieved in external process indicator immediately after removal from sterilizer then check internal process indicator before use. Refer to state regulations for any additional state requirements.

Laboratory Bur—Diamond Disc

Function ▶ To contour or cut models in the laboratory

Characteristic ▶ Single- or double-sided cutting edge

Practice Note ▶ Laboratory Bur—Diamond Disc is inserted and secured in a slow-speed handpiece with a straight attachment.

Sterilization Notes ▶ Laboratory Bur—Diamond Disc, when used on any patient's appliances must be precleaned, either, placed in a sterilizing pouch with an internal process indicator, sealed, then sterilized OR wrapped with an internal process indicator inside and secured on the outside with process indicator tape, then sterilized. Verify appropriate color change has been achieved in external process indicator immediately after removal from sterilizer then check internal process indicator before use. Refer to state regulations for any additional state requirements.

Magnetic Bur Block with Burs

Function ▶ To be used on dental tray setups

Characteristics ▶ Magnetic to hold burs in place
Holds friction grip and latch-type burs
Variety of shapes and sizes available
Various colors available to coordinate with color of tray

Practice Note ▶ Magnetic Bur Blocks with Burs are used on most restorative tray setups.

Sterilization Notes ▶ Magnetic Bur Block with Burs must be precleaned, either, placed in a sterilizing pouch with an internal process indicator, sealed, then sterilized OR wrapped with an internal process indicator inside and secured on the outside with process indicator tape, then sterilized. Verify appropriate color change has been achieved in external process indicator immediately after removal from sterilizer then check internal process indicator before treatment. Refer to state regulations for any additional state requirements.

Dental Dam Instruments

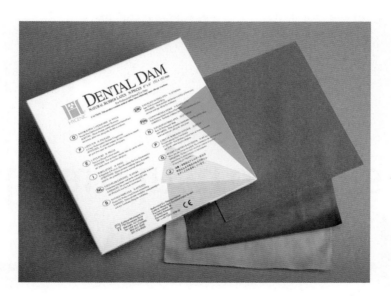

Dental Dam

Function ▶ To isolate teeth for dental procedures

Characteristics ▶ Sizes—4 × 4, 5 × 5, 6 × 6, or continuous roll
Gauge or thickness—Thin, medium, heavy
Colors—Gray, green, blue, pastels
Latex free—Purple

Practice Notes ▶ Latex-free Dental Dam (purple) is used for patients who have latex allergy.

Sterilization Notes ▶ Dental Dam should be disposed of in garbage. Single use only.

■INSTRUMENT Dental Dam Stamp

Function ▶ To mark holes on dental dam

Characteristics ▶ Has 32 dots that represent the adult dentition
Used as guide for punching holes in correct position

Practice Notes ▶ The oral cavity is examined before holes are marked and punched to adjust positioning to the patient's specific dentition.

Sterilization Notes ▶ Dental Dam Stamp should be disinfected according to the manufacturer's recommendation.

Place dam on top of template: mark with pen.

MAXILLARY

MANDIBULAR

THE HYGENIC CORPORATION   **6X6 DAM TEMPLATE**

Dental Dam Template

Function ▶ To use as a guide for marking and punching holes in correct position on dental dam

Characteristics ▶ Made of durable plastic

Has 32 dots that represent the adult dentition

Practice Notes ▶ The oral cavity is examined before holes are marked and punched to adjust positioning to the patient's specific dentition.

The dental dam is placed on the template, and the points where holes should be punched are marked with a pen.

Sterilization Notes ▶ Dental Dam Template should be disinfected according to the manufacturer's recommendation.

Dental Dam Punch

Function ▶ To punch holes in dental dam for each individual tooth

Characteristics ▶ Designated hole size for each tooth for permanent
dentition:

No. 5—Anchor tooth (largest)

No. 4—Molars

No. 3—Premolars

No. 2—Maxillary central and laterals, maxillary
and mandibular cuspids

No. 1—Mandibular central and laterals (smallest)

Practice Notes ▶ The oral cavity is examined before holes are punched to accommodate the patient's specific
dentition.

A space of 3 to 3.5 mm is maintained between holes.

Sterilization Notes ▶ Dental Dam Punch must be precleaned open and unlocked, placed in an open and unlocked
position either in a sterilizing pouch with an internal process indicator, sealed, then
sterilized OR wrapped with an internal process indicator inside and secured on the outside
with process indicator tape, then sterilized. Verify appropriate color change has been
achieved in external process indicator immediately after removal from sterilizer then check
internal process indicator before treatment. Refer to state regulations for any additional state
requirements.

▪INSTRUMENT Dental Dam Forceps

Function ▶ To place dental dam clamp on tooth and to remove clamp after procedure

Characteristics ▶ Beaks on forceps fit into dental dam clamp.
Forceps open with spring motion.
Bar between handle holds forceps in place while clamp is seated.

Practice Note ▶ Squeeze handles on dental dam forceps to open working end.

Sterilization Notes ▶ Dental Dam Forceps must be precleaned open and unlocked, placed in an open and unlocked position either in a sterilizing pouch with an internal process indicator, sealed, then sterilized OR wrapped with an internal process indicator inside and secured on the outside with process indicator tape, then sterilized. Verify appropriate color change has been achieved in external process indicator immediately after removal from sterilizer then check internal process indicator before treatment. Refer to state regulations for any additional state requirements. For safety, dental floss (ligature tie) must be attached to each dental clamp before each use to allow for retrieval of clamp if dislodged and patient inhales or swallows.

Dental Dam Clamp

Function ▶ To anchor and stabilize dental dam

Characteristics ▶ Parts:

1 Bow: Placed toward distal part of tooth
2 Jaws: Have four prongs that secure clamp on tooth
3 Holes: On jaws; designated for beaks on forceps to place clamp on tooth
4 Prongs: Designed to secure clamp on cervical part of tooth, beyond the height of contour
5 Winged clamps: Have extension of metal on jaws to hold dental dam away for better visibility (Wingless clamps do not have extra extension of metal.)

For safety, dental floss (ligature tie) must be attached to each dental clamp before each use to allow for retrieval of clamp if dislodged and patient inhales or swallows.

Sterilization Notes ▶ Dental Dam Clamp must be precleaned, either, placed in a sterilizing pouch with an internal process indicator, sealed, then sterilized OR wrapped with an internal process indicator inside and secured on the outside with process indicator tape, then sterilized. Verify appropriate color change has been achieved in external process indicator immediately after removal from sterilizer then check internal process indicator before treatment. Refer to state regulations for any additional state requirements.

∎INSTRUMENT Anterior Clamp

Function ▶ To anchor and stabilize dental dam

Characteristics ▶ Used only on anterior teeth
Example: Wingless clamp

Range of sizes available

Practice Notes ▶ Anterior clamp is used on a dental dam setup for restorative and endodontic procedures.

For safety, dental floss (ligature tie) must be attached to each dental clamp before each use to allow for retrieval of clamp if dislodged and patient inhales or swallows.

Sterilization Notes ▶ Anterior Clamp must be precleaned, either, placed in a sterilizing pouch with an internal process indicator, sealed, then sterilized OR wrapped with an internal process indicator inside and secured on the outside with process indicator tape, then sterilized. Verify appropriate color change has been achieved in external process indicator immediately after removal from sterilizer then check internal process indicator before treatment. Refer to state regulations for any additional state requirements.

Premolar Clamp

Function ▶ To anchor and stabilize dental dam

Characteristics ▶ Clamp used is determined by tooth size.
Range of sizes available
Variety of styles
Examples:

1 Wingless clamp
2 Winged clamp

Practice Notes ▶ Premolar Clamp is used on a dental dam setup for restorative and endodontic procedures. For safety, dental floss (ligature tie) must be attached to each dental clamp before each use to allow for retrieval of clamp if dislodged and patient inhales or swallows.

Sterilization Notes ▶ Premolar Clamp must be precleaned, either, placed in a sterilizing pouch with an internal process indicator, sealed, then sterilized OR wrapped with an internal process indicator inside and secured on the outside with process indicator tape, then sterilized. Verify appropriate color change has been achieved in external process indicator immediately after removal from sterilizer then check internal process indicator before treatment. Refer to state regulations for any additional state requirements.

Universal Clamp—Maxillary

Function ▶ To anchor and stabilize dental dam

Characteristics ▶ Used on right or left posterior molars
Range of sizes available
Variety of styles
Examples:

1 Wingless clamp
2 Winged clamp

Practice Notes ▶ Maxillary Clamp is used on a dental dam setup for restorative and endodontic procedures. For safety, dental floss (ligature tie) must be attached to each dental clamp before each use to allow for retrieval of clamp if dislodged and patient inhales or swallows.

Sterilization Notes ▶ Universal Maxillary Clamp must be precleaned, either, placed in a sterilizing pouch with an internal process indicator, sealed, then sterilized OR wrapped with an internal process indicator inside and secured on the outside with process indicator tape, then sterilized. Verify appropriate color change has been achieved in external process indicator immediately after removal from sterilizer then check internal process indicator before treatment. Refer to state regulations for any additional state requirements.

Universal Clamp—Mandibular

Function ▶ To anchor and stabilize dental dam

Characteristics ▶ Used on right or left posterior molars
Range of sizes available
Variety of styles
Examples:

1 Wingless clamp
2 Winged clamp

Practice Notes ▶ Mandibular Clamp is used on a dental dam setup for restorative and endodontic procedures. For safety, dental floss (ligature tie) must be attached to each dental clamp before each use to allow for retrieval of clamp if dislodged and patient inhales or swallows.

Sterilization Notes ▶ Universal Mandibular Clamp must be precleaned, either, placed in a sterilizing pouch with an internal process indicator, sealed, then sterilized OR wrapped with an internal process indicator inside and secured on the outside with process indicator tape, then sterilized. Verify appropriate color change has been achieved in external process indicator immediately after removal from sterilizer then check internal process indicator before treatment. Refer to state regulations for any additional state requirements.

Dental Dam Frame

Function ▶ To hold dental dam away from teeth

Characteristics ▶
1 Metal frame
2 Plastic frame

Plastic frame—May be left on during radiographic exposures
Various styles of frames available

Practice Notes ▶ Dental Dam Frame is used on a dental dam setup for
restorative and endodontic procedures.

Sterilization Notes ▶ Dental Dam Frame must be precleaned, either, placed in a
sterilizing pouch with an internal process indicator, sealed, then sterilized OR wrapped
with an internal process indicator inside and secured on the outside with process indicator
tape, then sterilized. Verify appropriate color change has been achieved in external process
indicator immediately after removal from sterilizer then check internal process indicator
before treatment. Refer to state regulations for any additional state requirements.

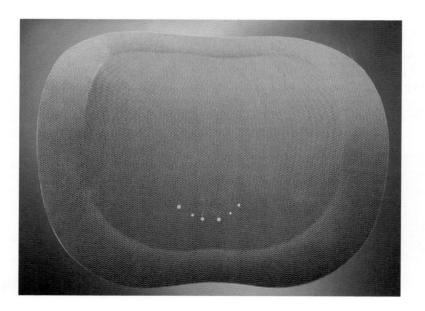

Preframed Dental Dam

Function ▶ To isolate teeth for dental procedures

Characteristics ▶ Frame is attached to dental dam
Dental dams may come pre-punched –
additional holes can be punched

Practice Note ▶ Dental Dam is latex free.
Dam adjusts to the side for easy access for
radiograph
Dam shown with secure ligatures to hold
Dental Dam in place instead of Dental Dam
clamp.

Sterilization Notes ▶ Dental Dam should be disposed of in
garbage. Single use only.

Dental Dam

LEFT (TOP TO BOTTOM)

Dental dam (latex free), dental floss, plastic dental dam frame, crown and bridge scissors (see Chapter 10)

RIGHT (TOP TO BOTTOM)

Beavertail burnisher used to invert Dental Dam (see Chapter 8), dental dam forceps, dental dam clamp with stabilizing ligature tie (dental floss), Dental Dam punch

Sterilization Notes ▶ Refer to each individual instrument for correct procedure for sterilization or disposal of instrument or material.

Amalgam Restorative Instruments

Tofflemire/Matrix Band Retainer

Function ▶ To hold and maintain stability of matrix band during condensation of restorative material for class II preparation

Characteristics ▶ Parts:

1 Guide slots: Straight slot; right and left slots for right or left quadrant

2 Diagonal slot: Slides up and down on spindle; matrix band is placed in slot, and spindle secures band in place; open slots are placed toward gingiva.

3 Spindle: Holds matrix band in retainer

4 Spindle pin: Stabilizes band in holder

5 Inner knob: Adjusts size of the loop of matrix band to fit around tooth and loosens band for removal

6 Outer knob: Positioned at end of spindle that tightens or loosens matrix band in retainer

Practice Notes ▶ Tofflemire Band Retainer is used on restorative tray setups.
The photo shown is for maxillary right quadrant and mandibular left quadrant.

Sterilization Notes ▶ Tofflemire Band Retainer must be precleaned open and unlocked, spindle should be disengaged, then, placed in an open and unlocked position either in a sterilizing pouch with an internal process indicator, sealed, then sterilized OR wrapped with an internal process indicator inside and secured on the outside with process indicator tape, then sterilized. Verify appropriate color change has been achieved in external process indicator immediately after removal from sterilizer then check internal process indicator before treatment. Refer to state regulations for any additional state requirements.

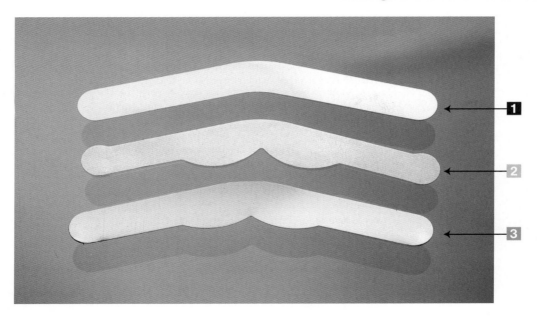

▪INSTRUMENT   Matrix Bands

Function ▸ To replace missing proximal wall or walls of cavity preparation for condensation of restorative material for class II preparations

Characteristics ▸ Variety of sizes, shapes, and thicknesses
Bands designed for specific types of restorations:

1 Universal band—For restorations on all posterior teeth except for teeth with deep cervical restorations—Example: MO, DO, MOD

2 Bands for teeth with deep cervical restorations—Example: Premolars that have a deep cervical restoration. Example: MO, DO, or MOD

3 Bands for larger teeth with deep cervical restorations—Example: Larger teeth such as Molars that have a deep cervical restoration. Example: MO, DO, MOD

Variety of pediatric bands available for primary teeth

Practice Note ▸ Matrix Bands are used on amalgam, composite, buildup, and temporary filling tray setups.

Sterilization Notes ▸ Matrix Bands should be disposed of in a sharps container, and/or local and state regulations should be followed. Single use only.

Matrix Band System

Function ▶ To replace missing proximal wall or walls of cavity preparation for condensation of restorative material for class II preparations

Characteristics ▶ Variety of matrix band systems (pictured: AutoMatrix)
Variety of sizes and shapes
Bands designed for specific teeth:

- Universal—Posterior teeth
- Molar—Larger molars
- Premolar
- Pediatric—Primary teeth

Practice Notes ▶ Tightening wrench is used to place, tighten, and loosen bands.
Removing pliers are used to remove bands.
Matrix Bands are used on amalgam, composite, buildup, and temporary filling tray setups.

Sterilization Notes ▶ Matrix Bands should be disposed of in sharps container, or local and state regulations should be followed. Single use only. Matrix Band Instruments should be placed in an open and unlocked position either in a sterilizing pouch with an internal process indicator, sealed, then sterilized OR wrapped with an internal process indicator inside and secured on the outside with process indicator tape, then sterilized. Verify appropriate color change has been achieved in external process indicator immediately after removal from sterilizer then check internal process indicator before treatment. Refer to state regulations for any additional state requirements.

Wooden Wedges

Function ▶ To hold matrix band in place along gingival margin of class II, class III, or class IV preparation

Characteristics ▶ Wood or plastic
Triangular, round, or anatomical shapes (shown in picture)
Variety of sizes and shapes available to accommodate embrasure area

Practice Notes ▶ Wedges are placed in gingival embrasure area usually on the lingual.
Wedges are always set up with all types of matrix band systems for class II, class III, or class IV restorations.

Sterilization Notes ▶ Wooden Wedges should be disposed of in the garbage.
Single use only.

■INSTRUMENT Liner Applicator

Function ▶ To place dental liner material (such as calcium hydroxide or glass ionomer) in cavity preparation

Characteristics ▶ Short or long handle
Single or double ended

Practice Notes ▶ Liner Applicator is used on amalgam, composite, crown and bridge, and temporary filling tray setups.
Also referred to as a Dycal instrument

Sterilization Notes ▶ Liner Applicator must be precleaned, either, placed in a sterilizing pouch with an internal process indicator, sealed, then sterilized OR wrapped with an internal process indicator inside and secured on the outside with process indicator tape, then sterilized. Verify appropriate color change has been achieved in external process indicator immediately after removal from sterilizer then check internal process indicator before treatment. Refer to state regulations for any additional state requirements.

Woodson

Functions ▶ To carry and place temporary restorative material for cavity preparation—Paddle end
To condense restorative material—Plugger end
To carry (paddle end) and condense a base (Plugger end)

Characteristics ▶ Double ended
Range of sizes available:

1. Plugger end available in variety of sizes
2. Paddle end available in different angles, sizes

Practice Notes ▶ Woodson is used on amalgam, composite, crown and bridge, temporary filling, and provisional crown tray setups.

Sterilization Notes ▶ Woodson must be precleaned, either, placed in a sterilizing pouch with an internal process indicator, sealed, then sterilized OR wrapped with an internal process indicator inside and secured on the outside with process indicator tape, then sterilized. Verify appropriate color change has been achieved in external process indicator immediately after removal from sterilizer then check internal process indicator before treatment. Refer to state regulations for any additional state requirements.

▪INSTRUMENT Amalgamator and Amalgam Capsule

Functions ▶ To mix alloy and mercury into amalgam in a capsule
To mix other types of restorative materials in a capsule
To mix precapsulated permanent and temporary cements

Characteristics ▶ **1** Amalgamator
2 Preloaded amalgam capsules contain alloy, mercury, and pestle to aid mixing:

- Various types of capsules are available; they are activated manually by twisting or pushing or using a capsule activator.

Thin membrane separates materials until mixing occurs.

Practice Notes ▶ The process of mixing is called amalgamation or trituration.
The mixing time recommended by the manufacturer should be used.

Sterilization Notes ▶ Capsules must be disposed of in the garbage, or state regulations must be followed. Single use only. Excess amalgam must be disposed of as amalgam waste material. Refer to local and state regulations for disposal. Amalgamator should be handled with overgloves or precleaned and disinfected according to the manufacturer's recommendation.

Amalgam Well

Functions ▶
To hold amalgam before it is placed in preparation
To hold amalgam while loading amalgam carrier

Characteristic ▶
Metal (shown in picture), plastic, or glass

Practice Notes ▶
Amalgam Well is used on the amalgam tray setup.

Sterilization Notes ▶
Amalgam Well must be precleaned, either, placed in a sterilizing pouch with an internal process indicator, sealed, then sterilized OR wrapped with an internal process indicator inside and secured on the outside with process indicator tape, then sterilized. Verify appropriate color change has been achieved in external process indicator immediately after removal from sterilizer then check internal process indicator before treatment. Refer to state regulations for any additional state requirements. Excess amalgam must be disposed of as amalgam waste material. Refer to local and state regulations for disposal.

Amalgam Carrier

Function ▶ To carry and dispense amalgam into cavity preparation

Characteristics ▶ Single or double ended:

1 Double ended—One small end and one large end
2 Single ended—Plunger style

The inside of the hollow tubes is coated with metal or Teflon.

Practice Notes ▶ Amalgam is packed in hollow tubes and then transferred to the cavity preparation. Amalgam sticks in the carrier if it is not released immediately after the tubes are filled. Amalgam Carrier is used exclusively on amalgam tray setups.

Sterilization Notes ▶ Amalgam Carrier must be precleaned, either, placed in a sterilizing pouch with an internal process indicator, sealed, then sterilized OR wrapped with an internal process indicator inside and secured on the outside with process indicator tape, then sterilized. Verify appropriate color change has been achieved in external process indicator immediately after removal from sterilizer then check internal process indicator before treatment. Refer to state regulations for any additional state requirements. Excess amalgam must be disposed of as amalgam waste material. Refer to local and state regulations for disposal.

Condenser (Plugger)—Smooth and Serrated

Functions ▶ To pack and condense amalgam into cavity preparation
To pack and condense other restorative materials
To pack and condense temporary filling material

Characteristics ▶
1 Smooth end small
2 Smooth end large
3 Serrated ends

Round, flat, or diamond shaped
Single or double ended
• Double ended—One small end and one large end
Back action condenser available with right-angle working ends—
Accommodates difficult areas
Range of sizes available

Practice Notes ▶ Smooth and Serrated Condensers are used on amalgam, composite, and temporary filling tray setups.

Sterilization Notes ▶ Smooth and Serrated Condensers must be precleaned, either, placed in a sterilizing pouch with an internal process indicator, sealed, then sterilized OR wrapped with an internal process indicator inside and secured on the outside with process indicator tape, then sterilized. Verify appropriate color change has been achieved in external process indicator immediately after removal from sterilizer then check internal process indicator before treatment. Refer to state regulations for any additional state requirements. Excess amalgam must be disposed of as amalgam waste material. Refer to local and state regulations for disposal.

Interproximal Condenser

Functions ▶ To pack and condense amalgam into interproximal areas
of cavity preparation
To pack and condense other restorative materials

Characteristics ▶ Ends shaped to fit mesial or distal areas of cavity
preparation
Smooth or serrated ends
Range of sizes available

Practice Note ▶ Interproximal Condenser is used on amalgam, composite,
and temporary filling tray setups.

Sterilization Notes ▶ Interproximal Condenser must be precleaned, either, placed in a sterilizing pouch with
an internal process indicator, sealed, then sterilized OR wrapped with an internal process
indicator inside and secured on the outside with process indicator tape, then sterilized.
Verify appropriate color change has been achieved in external process indicator immediately
after removal from sterilizer then check internal process indicator before treatment. Refer to
state regulations for any additional state requirements. Excess amalgam must be disposed of
as amalgam waste material. Refer to local and state regulations for disposal.

Burnishers—Football, Ball, and Acorn

Functions ▶
To smooth amalgam after condensing
To contour matrix band before placement
To perform initial shaping of amalgam
To burnish restorative material
To burnish temporary filling material

Characteristics ▶
1 Football burnisher
2 Ball burnisher
3 Acorn burnisher

Single or double ended–some double ended burnishers may have two different types of burnishers

Practice Note ▶
Football, Ball, and Acorn Burnishers are used on amalgam, composite, and temporary filling tray setups.

Sterilization Notes ▶
Football, Ball, and Acorn Burnishers must be precleaned, either, placed in a sterilizing pouch with an internal process indicator, sealed, then sterilized OR wrapped with an internal process indicator inside and secured on the outside with process indicator tape, then sterilized. Verify appropriate color change has been achieved in external process indicator immediately after removal from sterilizer then check internal process indicator before treatment. Refer to state regulations for any additional state requirements. Excess amalgam must be disposed of as amalgam waste material. Refer to local and state regulations for disposal.

T-Ball Burnisher

Functions ▶ To smooth amalgam after condensing
To contour matrix band before placement
To begin shaping of amalgam
To burnish restorative materials
To burnish temporary filling material

Characteristic ▶ Single ended

Practice Notes ▶ T-Ball Burnisher is used on amalgam, composite, and temporary filling tray setups.

Sterilization Notes ▶ T-Ball Burnisher must be precleaned, either, placed in a sterilizing pouch with an internal process indicator, sealed, then sterilized OR wrapped with an internal process indicator inside and secured on the outside with process indicator tape, then sterilized. Verify appropriate color change has been achieved in external process indicator immediately after removal from sterilizer then check internal process indicator before treatment. Refer to state regulations for any additional state requirements. Excess amalgam must be disposed of as amalgam waste material. Refer to local and state regulations for disposal.

■INSTRUMENT Beavertail Burnisher

Functions ▶
To smooth amalgam after condensing
To perform initial shaping and/or carving of amalgam
To invert dental dam (refer to dental dam tray setup in Chapter 7)
To burnish restorative materials
To burnish temporary filling material

Characteristic ▶ Single or double ended

Practice Note ▶ Beavertail Burnisher is used on amalgam, temporary filling, and dental dam tray setups.

Sterilization Notes ▶ Beavertail Burnisher must be precleaned, either, placed in a sterilizing pouch with an internal process indicator, sealed, then sterilized OR wrapped with an internal process indicator inside and secured on the outside with process indicator tape, then sterilized. Verify appropriate color change has been achieved in external process indicator immediately after removal from sterilizer then check internal process indicator before treatment. Refer to state regulations for any additional state requirements. Excess amalgam must be disposed of as amalgam waste material. Refer to local and state regulations for disposal.

Tanner Carver

Functions ▶ To carve occlusal anatomy into amalgam restorations
To carve occlusal anatomy in other restorative and
temporary filling materials

Characteristics ▶ Double ended—Two ends shaped differently
Ends shaped differently from those of discoid-cleoid carver

Practice Notes ▶ Tanner Carver is used on amalgam and temporary filling tray
setups.

Sterilization Notes ▶ Tanner Carver must be precleaned, either, placed in a
sterilizing pouch with an internal process indicator, sealed,
then sterilized OR wrapped with an internal process
indicator inside and secured on the outside with process indicator tape, then sterilized.
Verify appropriate color change has been achieved in external process indicator immediately
after removal from sterilizer then check internal process indicator before treatment. Refer to
state regulations for any additional state requirements. Excess amalgam must be disposed of
as amalgam waste material. Refer to local and state regulations for disposal.

Discoid-Cleoid Carver

Functions ▸ To carve occlusal anatomy into amalgam restorations

To carve occlusal anatomy in other restorative and temporary filling materials

Characteristics ▸ Double ended—Two ends shaped differently:

1 Discoid end—Disc shaped
2 Cleoid end—Pointed

Ends shaped differently from those of Tanner carver

Practice Notes ▸ Discoid-Cleoid Carver is used on amalgam and temporary filling tray setups.

Sterilization Notes ▸ Discoid-Cleoid Carver must be precleaned, either, placed in a sterilizing pouch with an internal process indicator, sealed, then sterilized OR wrapped with an internal process indicator inside and secured on the outside with process indicator tape, then sterilized. Verify appropriate color change has been achieved in external process indicator immediately after removal from sterilizer then check internal process indicator before treatment. Refer to state regulations for any additional state requirements. Excess amalgam must be disposed of as amalgam waste material. Refer to local and state regulations for disposal.

Hollenback and Half-Hollenback Carvers

Functions ▶ To contour and carve occlusal and interproximal anatomy in amalgam restorations

To contour and carve occlusal and interproximal anatomy in other restorative and temporary filling materials

Characteristics ▶ **1** Hollenback

2 Half-Hollenback—Half the size of Hollenback carver

Double ended—Working ends protrude at different angles.

Practice Note ▶ Hollenback and Half-Hollenback Carvers are used on amalgam, composite, and temporary filling tray setups.

Sterilization Notes ▶ Hollenback and Half-Hollenback Carvers must be precleaned, either, placed in a sterilizing pouch with an internal process indicator, sealed, then sterilized OR wrapped with an internal process indicator inside and secured on the outside with process indicator tape, then sterilized. Verify appropriate color change has been achieved in external process indicator immediately after removal from sterilizer then check internal process indicator before treatment. Refer to state regulations for any additional state requirements. Excess amalgam must be disposed of as amalgam waste material. Refer to local and state regulations for disposal.

Gold Carving Knife

Functions ▶ To trim interproximal amalgam restoration, recreating contour of proximal wall(s)
To trim interproximal restorations with other restorative materials, recreating contour of proximal wall(s)
To remove flash composite material from interproximal areas

Characteristics ▶ Single or double ended
Variety of designs
Interproximal carving knife-Different Styles available as shown above

Practice Notes ▶ Gold Carving Knife is used on amalgam and composite restorative tray setups.

Sterilization Notes ▶ Gold Carving Knife must be precleaned, either, placed in a sterilizing pouch with an internal process indicator, sealed, then sterilized OR wrapped with an internal process indicator inside and secured on the outside with process indicator tape, then sterilized. Verify appropriate color change has been achieved in external process indicator immediately after removal from sterilizer then check internal process indicator before treatment. Refer to state regulations for any additional state requirements. Excess amalgam must be disposed of as amalgam waste material. Refer to local and state regulations for disposal.

Articulating Paper Holder

■INSTRUMENT

Functions ▶ To hold articulating paper in place
To check centric and lateral occlusion

Characteristics ▶
1 Metal articulating paper holder
2 Disposable articulating paper holder

Articulating paper—blue (top) or red (bottom)
Paper variety—from thin to thick

Practice Notes ▶ Articulating Paper Holder and articulating paper are used on all restorative tray setups, including but not limited to amalgam, composite, fixed and removable prosthodontics, provisional crown, endodontics, orthodontic retainer delivery, and temporary filling tray setups.

Sterilization Notes ▶ Articulating Paper Holder (metal type) must be precleaned, either, placed in a sterilizing pouch with an internal process indicator, sealed, then sterilized OR wrapped with an internal process indicator inside and secured on the outside with process indicator tape, then sterilized. Verify appropriate color change has been achieved in external process indicator immediately after removal from sterilizer then check internal process indicator before treatment. Refer to state regulations for any additional state requirements. Disposable Articulating Paper Holder and Articulating Paper should be disposed of in the garbage. Single use only. Excess amalgam must be disposed of as amalgam waste material. Refer to local and state regulations for disposal.

Amalgam

TOP ROW (LEFT TO RIGHT)
Amalgam well, HVE tip, burs in bur block, amalgam carrier-plunger style (very top of tray)

BOTTOM ROW (LEFT TO RIGHT)
Mouth mirror, explorer, cotton forceps (pliers), spoon excavator, enamel hatchet, mesial gingival margin trimmer, distal gingival margin trimmer, small condenser, large condenser, acorn burnisher, Tanner carver, half-Hollenback carver, gold carving knife, Tofflemire, wooden wedges, crown and bridge scissors, articulating paper holder and articulating paper, liner applicator, dental floss, anesthetic aspirating syringe, air/water syringe tip

Sterilization Notes ▶ Refer to each individual picture for correct procedure for instrument sterilization or disposal of instrument or material. Refer to other chapters for additional instruments on this tray setup that are not included in this chapter.

Composite Restorative Instruments

INSTRUMENT Sectional Matrix System

Function ▶ To replace missing proximal wall of cavity preparation for placement of composite material or other restorative materials for class II restorations

Characteristics ▶ Variety of sizes and shapes to accommodate restoration:

1 Pediatric band—Primary molar

2 Small band—Premolar, small molar

3 Extended small band—Premolar, molar, with deep cervical restoration

4 Standard band—Molar restoration

5 Large band—Deep cervical restoration

6 Tension rings—Different sizes to accommodate restoration

Placed to secure band on proximal wall
Placed on tooth with dental dam forceps (Refer to page 170, Chapter 7)

Practice Notes ▶ Sectional Bands are used on amalgam, composite, buildup, and temporary filling tray setups.
Classes III and IV composite restorations use a clear Mylar matrix strip.

Sterilization Notes ▶ Sectional Bands should be disposed of in sharps container, or state regulations should be followed. Single use only. Tension rings must be precleaned, either, placed in a sterilizing pouch with an internal process indicator, sealed, then sterilized OR wrapped with an internal process indicator inside and secured on the outside with process indicator tape, then sterilized. Verify appropriate color change has been achieved in external process indicator immediately after removal from sterilizer then check internal process indicator before treatment. Refer to state regulations for any additional state requirements.

Applicator

Functions ▶ To apply conditioning, primer, and bonding material to cavity preparation
To use with bonding procedures, sealants, and orthodontic band brackets

Characteristics ▶ Types:

1 Disposable One-piece Applicator—Several colors available for application of different materials; working end bends; various styles, sizes

2 Microbrush Applicator—Disposable, various styles, sizes

Practice Notes ▶ Applicators are used on composite, sealant tray setups and any procedure involving etching, primers, and bonding materials.

Sterilization Notes ▶ Disposable Applicator(s) should be disposed of in the garbage. Single use only.

∎INSTRUMENT Well for Composite Material

Function ▶ To hold material: etchant, primers, bonding, and composite

Characteristics ▶
- **1** Disposable (pictured) or autoclavable
- **2** Well with protective light cover

Labels on each well—Designate different materials
Variety of styles and colors available

Practice Notes ▶ Wells are also used on a sealant tray setup and any procedure involving etching, primers, and bonding.

Sterilization Notes ▶ Disposable Wells should be disposed of in the garbage. Must be precleaned, either, placed in a sterilizing pouch with an internal process indicator, sealed, then sterilized OR wrapped with an internal process indicator inside and secured on the outside with process indicator tape, then sterilized. Verify appropriate color change has been achieved in external process indicator immediately after removal from sterilizer then check internal process indicator before treatment. Refer to state regulations for any additional state requirements. Refer to manufacturer's recommendations.

Composite Placement Instrument

Functions ▶ To carry composite material to the cavity preparation
To place, condense, and carve composite material in cavity preparation

Characteristics ▶
1 Plastic composite instrument—Plastic that can be sterilized

2 Metal composite instruments—Titanium nitride coating

Double ended
Different angles on ends
Ends shaped differently, one to accommodate initial placement of material (paddle end) and the other end to condense, contour, and carve material
Variety of sizes, shapes, and angles available

Practice Notes ▶ Composite Placement Instrument is used on composite tray setups.

Sterilization Notes ▶ Composite Placement Instrument must be precleaned, either, placed in a sterilizing pouch with an internal process indicator, sealed, then sterilized OR wrapped with an internal process indicator inside and secured on the outside with process indicator tape, then sterilized. Verify appropriate color change has been achieved in external process indicator immediately after removal from sterilizer then check internal process indicator before treatment. Refer to state regulations for any additional state requirements.

Composite Burnisher

Functions ▶ To form occlusal anatomy in composite restorations
To achieve final contouring of anatomy, pits, fissures, and grooves

Characteristics ▶ Double ended—Different angle on either end

1 Composite Burnisher: Titanium nitride coating—Creates hard, smooth, nonstick surface that resists scratching, sticking, or discoloration of composite material

2 Acorn Burnisher (for composite restorations):

Gold titanium nitride coating—Creates hard, smooth, nonstick surface that resists scratching, sticking, or discoloration of composite material

Practice Notes ▶ Composite Burnisher is used on composite tray setups.

Sterilization Notes ▶ Composite Burnisher must be precleaned, either, placed in a sterilizing pouch with an internal process indicator, sealed, then sterilized OR wrapped with an internal process indicator inside and secured on the outside with process indicator tape, then sterilized. Verify appropriate color change has been achieved in external process indicator immediately after removal from sterilizer then check internal process indicator before treatment. Refer to state regulations for any additional state requirements.

Curing Light—Battery Operated

Function ▶ To harden light-cured materials: bonding agents, composite, sealants, buildup material

Characteristics ▶ Battery operated—Includes battery charger with extra battery

Practice Notes ▶ Material must be cured in increments of 2 mm or less to ensure complete setting.
Refer to manufacturer's recommendation for curing time.

Sterilization Notes ▶ A testing device should be used to check the accuracy of the Curing Light. Protective sleeves are available for the curing lights. Preclean and disinfect the wand and light using disinfectant solution according to the manufacturer's recommendation.

Protective Shield for Curing Light

Function ▶ To protect eyes during curing stage of light-cured material

Characteristics ▶ Orange color—Blocks harmful light to operator/assistant and patient's eyes
Protective shields also available on curing light (see Curing Light, page 242)

1 Paddle Shield style
2 Protective eyeglasses available for operator, assistant, and patient

Practice Notes ▶ Protective Shield must be used with all curing lights.

Sterilization Notes ▶ Protective Shield, paddle, glasses must be precleaned and disinfected according to the manufacturer's recommendation.

LED and Halogen Radiometers

Functions ▶ To accurately test the visible light output for the LED
and halogen curing lights
To determine the accuracy of the LED and halogen
lights that cure dental materials

Characteristics ▶ White—Halogen Radiometer
Blue—LED Radiometer

Practice Notes ▶ Loss of output of the curing lights will affect the amount
of time needed to efficiently cure dental material.

Lights should be tested periodically to ensure lightbulb
and battery are working efficiently.

Sterilization Notes ▶ Refer to manufacturer's recommendation for disinfecting Radiometers.

Finishing Strip

Function ▶ To finish and smooth interproximal surface of restoration

Characteristics ▶ Abrasive textures available: synthetic or sandpaper material
Different grit consistencies available
Different grit consistency is on either end of strip—see color difference.

Practice Notes ▶ Synthetic Finishing Strip—No abrasive material in center of strip; helps avoid removal of tooth structure while inserting the finishing strip interproximally.
Finishing Strip is used on composite and amalgam tray setups.

Sterilization Notes ▶ Finishing Strip should be disposed of in the garbage. Single use only.

Composite Procedure—Class III and Class IV Composite Restorative

TOP ROW (FROM LEFT TO RIGHT)

High-volume evacuator (HVE) tip, well for composite material, burs and mandrel or discs in bur block, shade guide

BOTTOM ROW (FROM LEFT TO RIGHT)

Mouth mirror, explorer, cotton forceps (pliers), spoon excavator, composite placement instrument (titanium nitride coating), composite placement instrument (plastic), gold carving knife, liner applicator, three different colors of applicator brushes, wooden wedges, clear Mylar matrix strip and clamp to hold matrix, crown and bridge scissors, articulating paper holder and articulating paper, dental floss, anesthetic aspirating syringe, air/water syringe tip

Sterilization Notes ▶ Refer to each picture for correct procedure for instrument sterilization or disposal of material. Refer to other chapters for additional instruments on this tray setup that are not included in this chapter.

Composite Procedure—Class I, Class II, and Class V Composite Restorative

TOP ROW (LEFT TO RIGHT)

Articulating paper holder and articulating paper, well for composite material, shade guide

BOTTOM ROW (LEFT TO RIGHT)

Mouth mirror, explorer, cotton forceps (pliers), spoon excavator, composite placement instrument (titanium nitride coating), composite placement instrument (plastic), composite burnisher (gold–titanium nitride coating), gold carving knife, liner applicator, three different colors of applicator brushes, high-volume evacuator (HVE) tip, anesthetic syringe, dental damn forceps used for tension rings, (under forceps: matrix band, wooden wedges, tension rings, burs, mandrel/discs in bur block), dental floss, air/water syringe tip

BOTTOM OF TRAY

Finishing strip

Sterilization Notes ▶ Refer to each picture for correct procedure for instrument sterilization or disposal of material. Refer to other chapters for additional instruments on this tray setup that are not included in this chapter.

Fixed Prosthodontics Restorative Instruments

Facebow

Functions ▶ To establish the centric relationship of the maxillary teeth to the mandibular teeth

To establish the position of the teeth when the temporal mandibular joint is aligned correctly

Characteristics ▶ Recording and establishing the centric occlusion assists in fabricating fixed prosthodontic restorations

1 Apply compound tabs or dental impression material on bite fork

Recording and establishing the centric occlusion assists in fabricating fixed and removable prosthodontic appliances

Example: Crowns, bridges, partials and dentures.

Facebows are also used with orthodontic treatment assessment for mounting the impressions in correct occlusion

Practice Notes ▶ Facebow transfer applications are used in all phases of restorative dentistry.

Sterilization Notes ▶ Facebow outer appliances must be disinfected according to the manufacturer's recommendation. Bite Fork must be precleaned, either, placed in a sterilizing pouch with an internal process indicator, sealed, then sterilized OR wrapped with an internal process indicator inside and secured on the outside with process indicator tape, then sterilized. Verify appropriate color change has been achieved in external process indicator immediately after removal from sterilizer then check internal process indicator before treatment. Refer to state regulations for any additional state requirements.

Shade Guides/Digital Color Imaging

Functions ▸ To select a shade for permanent fixed restorations
Example: Crowns, veneers, bridges

To select a shade for removable appliances
Example: Partials, dentures

Characteristics ▸
1 Many different shade guides are available.
2 Many different digital or computerized shade guides are available.

Practice Notes ▸ Each tooth may have different shades: one for the gingival third, one for the body or middle third, and one for the incisal edge (usually needed for anteriors).

Sterilization Notes ▸ Shade Guides must be disinfected according to the manufacturer's recommendation.

Gingival Retraction Cord Instrument

Function ▶ To place gingival retraction cord in sulcus area after tooth is prepared for a crown and before final impressions are taken

Characteristics ▶ Smooth or serrated edges
Double ended—Different angle on each end
Variety of styles

Practice Notes ▶ Gingival Retraction Cord instrument is mainly used on crown and bridge tray setup unless gingiva needs to be retracted for a restorative procedure.

Sterilization Notes ▶ Gingival Retraction Cord Instrument must be precleaned, either, placed in a sterilizing pouch with an internal process indicator, sealed, then sterilized OR wrapped with an internal process indicator inside and secured on the outside with process indicator tape, then sterilized. Verify appropriate color change has been achieved in external process indicator immediately after removal from sterilizer then check internal process indicator before treatment. Refer to state regulations for any additional state requirements. Gingival retraction cord instrument should be disposed of in the garbage.

Crown and Bridge Scissors

Functions ▶
To trim aluminum temporary crowns on gingival side
To trim custom temporary crowns
To cut gingival retraction cord
To trim matrix bands
To cut dental dam septum

Characteristics ▶
Short cutting edges—can be straight or curved, narrow or wide
Variety of sizes

Practice Notes ▶
Crown and Bridge Scissors are used on other restorative tray setups.

Sterilization Notes ▶
Crown and Bridge Scissors must be precleaned open and unlocked, placed in an open and unlocked position either in a sterilizing pouch with an internal process indicator, sealed, then sterilized OR wrapped with an internal process indicator inside and secured on the outside with process indicator tape, then sterilized. Verify appropriate color change has been achieved in external process indicator immediately after removal from sterilizer then check internal process indicator before treatment. Refer to state regulations for any additional state requirements.

Contouring Pliers

Function ▶ To crimp and contour marginal edge of temporary crown or stainless steel crown

Characteristics ▶ Commonly used type: Johnson
Range of sizes available

Practice Notes ▶ Contouring Pliers are mainly used on crown and bridge tray setup.

Sterilization Notes ▶ Contouring Pliers must be precleaned open and unlocked, placed in an open and unlocked position either in a sterilizing pouch with an internal process indicator, sealed, then sterilized OR wrapped with an internal process indicator inside and secured on the outside with process indicator tape, then sterilized. Verify appropriate color change has been achieved in external process indicator immediately after removal from sterilizer then check internal process indicator before treatment. Refer to state regulations for any additional state requirements.

Provisional Crown–Removing Forceps

Function ▶ To remove provisional crown from tooth

Characteristic ▶ Range of sizes available

Practice Notes ▶ Provisional Crown–Removing Forceps are mainly used on crown and bridge tray setup.

Sterilization Notes ▶ Provisional Crown–Removing Forceps must be precleaned open and unlocked, placed in an open and unlocked position either in a sterilizing pouch with an internal process indicator, sealed, then sterilized OR wrapped with an internal process indicator inside and secured on the outside with process indicator tape, then sterilized. Verify appropriate color change has been achieved in external process indicator immediately after removal from sterilizer then check internal process indicator before treatment. Refer to state regulations for any additional state requirements.

CAD/CAM Machine

Functions ▶ To take a computer image of a tooth with an intraoral wand that connects to a computer
To construct the anatomy, gingival margins, occlusal and mesial/distal contacts of the crown on the computer
To send the information to the unit to construct the crown

Characteristics ▶ 1 Camera
2 CAD/CAM in-office system with attached camera

Crown is made of porcelain or other type materials.

Practice Notes ▶ The CAD/CAM machine allows the patient to have one appointment for preparing and seating a crown.

Sterilization Notes ▶ Barriers should be used for the intraoral wand. Barriers or overgloves should be used for manipulating the computer on the CAD/CAM-CEREC Machine. Otherwise, refer to the manufacturer's recommendation for disinfecting.

CAD/CA Milling Machine

Functions ▶ To mill the crown with the image taken from the camera that connects to the CAD/CAM

Characteristics ▶ 1 Milling machine
2 Ceramic blocks that are placed in the milling machine to fabricate the crown

As shown different shades are available.

Practice Notes ▶ CAD/CAM machine allows the patient to have one appointment for preparing and seating a crown.

Sterilization Notes ▶ Refer to manufacturer's recommendation for disinfecting.

Wooden Bite Stick

Function ▶ To seat permanent crown while patient bites in centric occlusion

Characteristics ▶ Soft wood
Range of sizes available

Practice Notes ▶ Wooden Bite Stick is primarily used on crown and bridge tray setup.
Other styles of biting devices to seat a crown are available including disposable devices

Sterilization Notes ▶ Wooden Bite Stick must be precleaned, either, placed in a sterilizing pouch with an internal process indicator, sealed, then sterilized OR wrapped with an internal process indicator inside and secured on the outside with process indicator tape, then sterilized. Verify appropriate color change has been achieved in external process indicator immediately after removal from sterilizer then check internal process indicator before treatment. Refer to state regulations for any additional state requirements. OR Wooden Bite Stick and other seating devices should be disposed of in the garbage.

Trial Crown Remover

Functions ▶ To remove permanent crown from tooth during try-in phase
To remove provisional crown

Characteristics ▶ Types:

1 Maxillary trial crown remover
2 Mandibular trial crown remover

Replaceable pads—Provide nonslipping, tight grip

Practice Notes ▶ Trial Crown Remover is mainly used on crown and
bridge tray setup.

Sterilization Notes ▶ Trial Crown Remover must be precleaned open and
unlocked, placed in an open and unlocked position
either in a sterilizing pouch with an internal process indicator, sealed, then sterilized OR
wrapped with an internal process indicator inside and secured on the outside with process
indicator tape, then sterilized. Verify appropriate color change has been achieved in external
process indicator immediately after removal from sterilizer then check internal process
indicator before treatment. Refer to state regulations for any additional state requirements.

Crown and Bridge Preparation

TOP ROW (LEFT TO RIGHT)
Gingival retraction cord, dental floss, burs in bur block

BOTTOM ROW (LEFT TO RIGHT)
Mouth mirror, explorer, cotton forceps (pliers), spoon excavator, curette, gingival retraction cord instrument, Woodson, crown and bridge scissors, flexible cement mixing spatula, articulating paper holder and articulating paper, provisional crown–removing forceps, anesthetic aspirating syringe, air/water syringe tip, high-volume evacuation (HVE) tip

Sterilization Notes ▶ Refer to each picture for correct procedure for instrument sterilization or disposal of material. Refer to other chapters for additional instruments on this tray setup that are not included in this chapter.

Crown and Bridge Cementation

TOP ROW (LEFT TO RIGHT)
Burs in bur block

BOTTOM ROW (LEFT TO RIGHT)
Mouth mirror, explorer, cotton forceps (pliers), spoon excavator, curette, Woodson, flexible cement mixing spatula, wooden bite stick, articulating paper holder and articulating paper, cotton rolls, provisional crown–removing forceps, dental floss (under provisional crown–removing forceps), trial crown remover (maxillary), air/water syringe tip, high-volume evacuation (HVE) tip

Sterilization Notes ▸ Refer to each picture for correct procedure for instrument sterilization or disposal of material. Refer to other chapters for additional instruments on this tray setup that are not included in this chapter.

Endodontic Instruments

Vitalometer/Pulp Tester

Function ▶ To test vitality of pulp in teeth

Characteristics ▶ Two types—Electronic and digital (digital readout)
Electric or battery operated

Practice Notes ▶ The tester sends an impulse of electric current to the pulp, causing a reaction.
The current is increased by small increments until the patient indicates feeling a sensation.
Toothpaste is applied to the tip of the electrode to conduct electricity.
The tip is placed on the surface part (facial or lingual) of a natural tooth.
Each root and pulp on the tooth is tested.
Vitalometer is used exclusively with endodontic tray setups.

Sterilization Notes ▶ Vitalometer tip must be precleaned, either, placed in a
sterilizing pouch with an internal process indicator, sealed, then
sterilized OR wrapped with an internal process indicator inside
and secured on the outside with process indicator tape, then
sterilized. Verify appropriate color change has been achieved
in external process indicator immediately after removal from
sterilizer then check internal process indicator before treatment.

Refer to state regulations for any additional state requirements. Barriers should be used on the
unit or the manufacturer's recommendation for disinfection of unit should be followed.

Endodontic Long-Shank Spoon Excavator

Function ▶ To reach deep into the canal to remove coronal pulp tissue, decay, and temporary cements

Characteristics ▶ Long shank to reach deep into cavity preparation
Double ended
Range of sizes available

Practice Notes ▶ Endodontic Long-Shank Spoon is used exclusively on endodontic tray setups.

Sterilization Notes ▶ Endodontic Long-Shank Spoon Excavator must be precleaned, either, placed in a sterilizing pouch with an internal process indicator, sealed, then sterilized OR wrapped with an internal process indicator inside and secured on the outside with process indicator tape, then sterilized. Verify appropriate color change has been achieved in external process indicator immediately after removal from sterilizer then check internal process indicator before treatment. Refer to state regulations for any additional state requirements.

Endodontic Explorer

Function ▶ To locate opening of small canal orifices for endodontic procedure

Characteristics ▶ Double ended
Working end—Longer than regular explorer to reach opening of canals

Practice Note ▶ Endodontic Explorer is used exclusively on endodontic tray setups.

Sterilization Notes ▶ Endodontic Explorer must be precleaned, either, placed in a sterilizing pouch with an internal process indicator, sealed, then sterilized OR wrapped with an internal process indicator inside and secured on the outside with process indicator tape, then sterilized. Verify appropriate color change has been achieved in external process indicator immediately after removal from sterilizer then check internal process indicator before treatment. Refer to state regulations for any additional state requirements.

■INSTRUMENT Endodontic Locking Forceps (Pliers)

Function ▸ To grasp and lock material for transfer into and out of oral cavity

Characteristic ▸ Similar to regular cotton forceps except for locking mechanism to secure material on the working end of the forceps (pliers)

Practice Note ▸ Endodontic Locking Forceps are used on endodontic tray setup and could also be used on restorative tray setups.

Sterilization Notes ▸ Endodontic Locking Forceps must be precleaned open and unlocked, placed in an open and unlocked position either in a sterilizing pouch with an internal process indicator, sealed, then sterilized OR wrapped with an internal process indicator inside and secured on the outside with process indicator tape, then sterilized. Verify appropriate color change has been achieved in external process indicator immediately after removal from sterilizer then check internal process indicator before treatment. Refer to state regulations for any additional state requirements.

▪INSTRUMENT Broach

Function ▶ To remove pulp tissue from canal(s)

Characteristics ▶ Working end—Barbed wire protrusions on shaft grab and remove vital or nonvital pulp fibers
Handles—Color coded according to size
Range of sizes—Diameter increases with size.

Practice Notes ▶ Endodontic Broach is used exclusively on endodontic tray setups.

Sterilization Notes ▶ Endodontic Broach must be disposed of in a sharps container. For single use only.

Endodontic File—K Type

Functions ▶ To clean inside walls of canal
To contour inner walls of canal

Characteristics ▶ Twisted design—More twists per millimeter than reamer
Used with push–pull motion
Handles—Color coded according to size
Range of sizes—To accommodate width of canal; diameter
increases with size.
Available in different lengths
Examples: 21 mm, 25 mm, 31 mm

Practice Note ▶ Endodontic File—K type is used exclusively on endodontic
tray setups.

Sterilization Notes ▶ Endodontic File—K Type must be precleaned, either, placed in a sterilizing pouch with
an internal process indicator, sealed, then sterilized OR wrapped with an internal process
indicator inside and secured on the outside with process indicator tape, then sterilized.
Verify appropriate color change has been achieved in external process indicator immediately
after removal from sterilizer then check internal process indicator before treatment. Refer to
state regulations for any additional state requirements. OR used File must be disposed of in
a sharps container. Rubber stopper on the file should be disposed of in the garbage.

Endodontic File—Hedstrom

Functions ▶ To clean inside walls of canal
To enlarge and smooth inner walls of canal

Characteristics ▶ Triangular cutting edge
Handles—Color coded according to size
Range of sizes—To accommodate width of canal; diameter increases with size.
Available in different lengths
Examples: 21 mm, 25 mm, 31 mm

Practice Note ▶ Endodontic File—Hedstrom is used exclusively on endodontic tray setups.

Sterilization Notes ▶ Endodontic File—Hedstrom must be precleaned, either, placed in a sterilizing pouch with an internal process indicator, sealed, then sterilized OR wrapped with an internal process indicator inside and secured on the outside with process indicator tape, then sterilized. Verify appropriate color change has been achieved in external process indicator immediately after removal from sterilizer then check internal process indicator before treatment. Refer to state regulations for any additional state requirements. OR used File must be disposed of in a sharps container. Rubber stopper on the file should be disposed of in the garbage.

∎INSTRUMENT Reamer

Functions ▶ To cut and smooth dentinal walls of canal
To enlarge inner walls of canal

Characteristics ▶ Twisted triangular cutting edge (similar to K-type file, but cutting edge is farther apart and has fewer twists per millimeter)
Used with twisting motion
Handles—Color coded according to size
Range of sizes—To accommodate width of canal; diameter increases with size.
Available in different lengths
Examples: 21 mm, 25 mm, 31 mm

Practice Note ▶ Reamer is used exclusively on endodontic tray setups.

Sterilization Notes ▶ Reamer must be precleaned, either, placed in a sterilizing pouch with an internal process indicator, sealed, then sterilized OR wrapped with an internal process indicator inside and secured on the outside with process indicator tape, then sterilized. Verify appropriate color change has been achieved in external process indicator immediately after removal from sterilizer then check internal process indicator before treatment. Refer to state regulations for any additional state requirements. Or used Reamer must be disposed of in a sharps container. Rubber stopper on the file should be disposed of in the garbage.

Endodontic Stoppers

Function ▶ To place onto an intracanal instrument such as a file or reamer to help determine length of canal

Characteristics ▶ Files or reamers are measured from stopper to apex of root to determine length of canal. (Radiographs also help determine length.)
Stoppers are made from rubber, silicone, or plastic.

Practice Notes ▶ Endodontic Stoppers are color coded to correspond to a particular file or reamer, or a single color of stopper is used for all files or reamers.
Endodontic Stoppers are used exclusively on endodontic tray setups.

Sterilization Notes ▶ Endodontic Stoppers should be disposed of in the garbage. Single use only.

Endodontic Stand

Functions ▶ To hold endodontic files and reamers
To measure endodontic files and reamers with millimeter ruler etched in container; may be measured from right or left side of stand

Characteristic ▶ Container closes with endodontic files and reamers for sterilization processes.

Practice Note ▶ Endodontic Stand is used exclusively with endodontic tray setups.

Sterilization Notes ▶ File or reamer in Endodontic Stand and endodontic stand must be precleaned, either, placed in a sterilizing pouch with an internal process indicator, sealed, then sterilized OR wrapped with an internal process indicator inside and secured on the outside with process indicator tape, then sterilized. Verify appropriate color change has been achieved in external process indicator immediately after removal from sterilizer then check internal process indicator before treatment. Refer to state regulations for any additional state requirements. Or used file or reamer must be disposed of in a sharps container. Rubber stopper on the file should be disposed of in the garbage. Single use only.

| ■INSTRUMENT | # Endodontic Millimeter Ruler |

Function ▶ To measure files, reamers, other instruments, and materials in millimeter increments

Characteristic ▶ Variety of designs

Practice Notes ▶ Endodontic Millimeter Ruler could be used in areas of dentistry other than on endodontic tray setups.

Sterilization Notes ▶ Endodontic Millimeter Ruler must be precleaned, either, placed in a sterilizing pouch with an internal process indicator, sealed, then sterilized OR wrapped with an internal process indicator inside and secured on the outside with process indicator tape, then sterilized. Verify appropriate color change has been achieved in external process indicator immediately after removal from sterilizer then check internal process indicator before treatment. Refer to state regulations for any additional state requirements.

▪INSTRUMENT Electronic Apex Locator

Function ▶ To electronically measure length of canal to apex of tooth

Characteristics ▶ Attaches to file or reamer and is placed in canal using dry or wet environment
Readout indicates length of canal—Tone or digital

Practice Note ▶ Electronic Apex Locator is used exclusively with endodontic tray setups.

Sterilization Notes ▶ Electronic Apex Locator device that enters patient's mouth must be precleaned, either, placed in a sterilizing pouch with an internal process indicator, sealed, then sterilized OR wrapped with an internal process indicator inside and secured on the outside with process indicator tape, then sterilized. Verify appropriate color change has been achieved in external process indicator immediately after removal from sterilizer then check internal process indicator before treatment. Refer to state regulations for any additional state requirements. Barriers should be used on the unit, or the manufacturer's recommendation for disinfection should be followed.

Gates Glidden Bur or Drill

Functions ▶ To enlarge walls of pulp chamber
To open canal orifice

Characteristics ▶ Long-shank bur
Elliptical or flame-shaped cutting edge
Latch type—Used with slow-speed contra-angle handpiece
(air driven or electric)
Range of sizes—Size identified by number of grooves on
shank
Two lengths—Shorter for posterior teeth, longer for
anterior teeth

Practice Note ▶ Gates Glidden Burs are used exclusively on endodontic tray setups.

Sterilization Notes ▶ Gates Glidden Bur or Drill must be precleaned, either, placed in a sterilizing pouch with
an internal process indicator, sealed, then sterilized OR wrapped with an internal process
indicator inside and secured on the outside with process indicator tape, then sterilized.
Verify appropriate color change has been achieved in external process indicator immediately
after removal from sterilizer then check internal process indicator before treatment. Refer to
state regulations for any additional state requirements. Or used Gates Glidden Bur must be
disposed of in a sharps container.

▪INSTRUMENT Endodontic Irrigating Syringe

Function ▶ To carry and dispense irrigating solution into canal for cleansing during débridement of canal

Characteristics ▶ Disposable
Two sizes—3 mL (pictured) and 12 mL

Practice Note ▶ Endodontic Irrigating Syringe could be used in areas of dentistry other than on endodontic tray setups.

Sterilization Notes ▶ Endodontic Irrigating Syringe should be disposed of in a sharps container. For single use only.

Sterile Absorbent Paper Points

Function ▶ To dry pulp chambers of canal—New points inserted repeatedly until pulp chamber is completely dry

Characteristics ▶ Size of point corresponds to width of canal
Range of sizes available

Practice Notes ▶ The length of the paper point is measured to ensure that it corresponds to the length of the canal.
Paper points are used exclusively on endodontic tray setups.

Sterilization Notes ▶ Sterile Absorbent Paper Points should be disposed of in the garbage. Single use only.

Gutta-Percha

Function ▶ To fill pulp chamber after completion of canal preparation (called obturation)

Characteristics ▶ Solid at room temperature; becomes soft and pliable when heated

May be heated in a cartridge and then dispensed into canal

Range of sizes—To correspond to size of canal

Practice Notes ▶ Endodontic sealer, a cement material, is used with gutta-percha for final sealing of the canal.

Gutta-Percha is used exclusively on an endodontic tray setup.

Sterilization Notes ▶ Gutta-Percha should be disposed of in the garbage.

Lentulo Spiral

Function ▶ To place endodontic sealer or cement in canal for final seal before placement of gutta-percha

Characteristic ▶ Latch-type shank—Used with slow-speed contra-angled handpiece (air driven or electric)

Practice Note ▶ Lentulo Spiral is used exclusively on endodontic tray setups.

Sterilization Notes ▶ Lentulo Spiral must be precleaned, either, placed in a sterilizing pouch with an internal process indicator, sealed, then sterilized OR wrapped with an internal process indicator inside and secured on the outside with process indicator tape, then sterilized. Verify appropriate color change has been achieved in external process indicator immediately after removal from sterilizer then check internal process indicator before treatment. Refer to state regulations for any additional state requirements. Or used lentulo spiral must be disposed of in a sharps container.

Gutta-Percha Warming Unit

Functions ▶ To heat gutta-percha outside the mouth before use
To inject heated gutta-percha in thermoplastic state into prepared canals

Characteristics ▶ Gutta-percha pellets—Used to load unit
Delivery system—Needle attaches to gun delivering gutta-percha into canal

Practice Notes ▶ Temperature of the gutta-percha in the unit can be adjusted to control the viscosity of the material.
Gutta-Percha warming unit is used exclusively with endodontic tray setups.

Sterilization Notes ▶ Gutta-Percha Warming Unit needle attached to the gutta-percha warming unit gun must be precleaned, either, placed in a sterilizing pouch with an internal process indicator, sealed, then sterilized OR wrapped with an internal process indicator inside and secured on the outside with process indicator tape, then sterilized. Verify appropriate color change has been achieved in external process indicator immediately after removal from sterilizer then check internal process indicator before treatment. Refer to state regulations for any additional state requirements. Or needle must be disposed of in a sharps container. Gutta-percha warming unit must be disinfected according to the manufacturer's recommendation.

▪INSTRUMENT Endodontic Spreader

Functions ▶
To help condense gutta-percha laterally in canal
To use for final filling of canal

Characteristics ▶
Pointed tip
Working end—Has rings in millimeter increments
Two handle styles—Conventional (pictured), finger spreader
Range of sizes—To correspond to size of canal

Practice Note ▶
Endodontic Spreader is used exclusively on endodontic tray setups.

Sterilization Notes ▶
Endodontic Spreader must be precleaned, either, placed in a sterilizing pouch with an internal process indicator, sealed, then sterilized OR wrapped with an internal process indicator inside and secured on the outside with process indicator tape, then sterilized. Verify appropriate color change has been achieved in external process indicator immediately after removal from sterilizer then check internal process indicator before treatment. Refer to state regulations for any additional state requirements.

Endodontic Plugger

Functions ▶ To help condense gutta-percha vertically in canal
To use for final filling of canal

Characteristics ▶ Flat tip for condensing gutta-percha
Working end—Has rings in millimeter increments
Two handle styles—Conventional (pictured), finger spreader
Range of sizes—To correspond to size of canal

Practice Note ▶ Endodontic Plugger is used exclusively on endodontic tray setups.

Sterilization Notes ▶ Endodontic Plugger must be precleaned, either, placed in a
sterilizing pouch with an internal process indicator, sealed, then
sterilized OR wrapped with an internal process indicator inside and
secured on the outside with process indicator tape, then sterilized.
Verify appropriate color change has been achieved in external
process indicator immediately after removal from sterilizer then
check internal process indicator before treatment. Refer to state
regulations for any additional state requirements.

Glick Instrument

Functions ▶ To condense gutta-percha into endodontically prepared teeth, using plugger end
To sever excess gutta-percha after plugger end is heated
To carry and place material into tooth, using paddle end

Characteristics ▶ Double ended:

1 Plugger end—May have rings in millimeter increments
2 Paddle end

Practice Note ▶ Glick Instrument is used exclusively on endodontic tray setups.

Sterilization Notes ▶ Glick Instrument must be precleaned, either, placed in a sterilizing pouch with an internal process indicator, sealed, then sterilized OR wrapped with an internal process indicator inside and secured on the outside with process indicator tape, then sterilized. Verify appropriate color change has been achieved in external process indicator immediately after removal from sterilizer then check internal process indicator before treatment. Refer to state regulations for any additional state requirements.

Peso File

Functions ▶ To prepare canal for endodontic post
To remove portion of gutta-percha sealed in canal to make room for endodontic post

Characteristics ▶ Parallel cutting edges
Latch-type shank—Used with slow-speed contra-angle handpiece (air driven or electric)
Range of sizes—Size identified by number of grooves on shank

Practice Note ▶ Peso File is used exclusively on endodontic tray setups.

Sterilization Notes ▶ Peso File must be precleaned, either, placed in a sterilizing pouch with an internal process indicator, sealed, then sterilized OR wrapped with an internal process indicator inside and secured on the outside with process indicator tape, then sterilized. Verify appropriate color change has been achieved in external process indicator immediately after removal from sterilizer then check internal process indicator before treatment. Refer to state regulations for any additional state requirements. Or used peso file must be disposed of in a sharps container.

∎INSTRUMENT # Micro Retro Amalgam Carrier

Function ▶ To carry amalgam to surgical site of apicoectomy

Characteristics ▶ Very small—To accommodate retro fills for apicoectomy
Surgical apicoectomy procedure is performed, if needed, after an endodontic procedure is completed.

Practice Note ▶ Micro Retro Amalgam Carrier is used with a surgical tray setup for an apicoectomy.

Sterilization Notes ▶ Micro Retro Amalgam Carrier must be precleaned, either, placed in a sterilizing pouch with an internal process indicator, sealed, then sterilized OR wrapped with an internal process indicator inside and secured on the outside with process indicator tape, then sterilized. Verify appropriate color change has been achieved in external process indicator immediately after removal from sterilizer then check internal process indicator before treatment. Refer to state regulations for any additional state requirements.

Micro Retro Mouth Mirror

Function ▶ To view surgical site of apicoectomy retro fill

Characteristics ▶ Very small—To accommodate retro fills for apicoectomy
Smaller sizes available

Practice Note ▶ Micro Retro Mouth Mirror is used with a surgical tray setup for an apicoectomy.

Sterilization Notes ▶ Micro Retro Mouth Mirror must be precleaned, either, placed in a sterilizing pouch with an internal process indicator, sealed, then sterilized OR wrapped with an internal process indicator inside and secured on the outside with process indicator tape, then sterilized. Verify appropriate color change has been achieved in external process indicator immediately after removal from sterilizer then check internal process indicator before treatment. Refer to state regulations for any additional state requirements.

Opening a Tooth for Endodontic Therapy

TOP ROW (LEFT TO RIGHT)

Millimeter ruler with finger ring; coarse, medium, and fine absorbent sterile paper points; burs in bur block

BOTTOM ROW (LEFT TO RIGHT)

Mouth mirror, endodontic explorer, endodontic locking forceps, endodontic long-shank spoon excavator, Glick instrument, Woodson, endodontic locking forceps (extra), irrigating disposable syringe, scissors, broaches, endodontic K-type file with color-coded rubber stops, anesthetic aspirating syringe, air/water syringe tip, high-volume evacuation (HVE) tip

Sterilization Notes ► Refer to each picture for correct procedure for instrument sterilization or disposal of instrument or material. Refer to other chapters for additional instruments on this tray setup that are not included in this chapter.

Sealing a Tooth for Endodontic Therapy

TOP ROW (LEFT TO RIGHT)

Millimeter ruler with finger ring; gutta-percha in vials—assorted sizes; coarse, medium, fine absorbent sterile paper points; burs in bur block

BOTTOM ROW (LEFT TO RIGHT)

Mouth mirror, endodontic explorer, endodontic locking forceps, endodontic long-shank spoon excavator, endodontic spreader, endodontic plugger, Glick instrument, Woodson, endodontic locking cotton forceps (extra), irrigating disposable syringe, scissors, endodontic K-type file with color-coded rubber stops, anesthetic aspirating syringe, air/water syringe tip, high-volume evacuation (HVE) tip

Sterilization Notes ▶ Refer to each picture for correct procedure for instrument sterilization or disposal of instrument or material. Refer to other chapters for additional instruments on this tray setup that are not included in this chapter.

Hygiene Instruments

Universal Curettes (Curets)

Functions ▶ To remove deposits and stains from teeth

To remove soft tissue lining of periodontal pocket and root planing

Characteristics ▶ Blade—Two cutting edges, rounded toe, rounded back; at 90-degree angle to lower shank

Flexible or rigid shank; length varies to accommodate clinical crown of tooth

Single or double ended

Range of sizes

Curette named by designer:

1 Barnhart ½
2 Ratcliff ⅜

Practice Note ▶ Universal Curettes are used on hygiene, periodontal, and operative tray setups.

Sterilization Notes ▶ Universal Curettes must be precleaned, either, placed in a sterilizing pouch with an internal process indicator, sealed, then sterilized OR wrapped with an internal process indicator inside and secured on the outside with process indicator tape, then sterilized. Verify appropriate color change has been achieved in external process indicator immediately after removal from sterilizer then check internal process indicator before treatment. Refer to state regulations for any additional state requirements.

∎INSTRUMENT Universal Curettes (Curet)

Functions ▶ To scale supragingival and subgingival surfaces
To remove deposits and stains from teeth
To remove soft tissue lining of periodontal pocket and root planing

Characteristics ▶ Blade—Two cutting edges, rounded toe, rounded back; at 90-degree angle to lower shank
Flexible or rigid shank; length varies to accommodate clinical crown of tooth
Single or double ended
Range of sizes
Curette named by designer:

1 UC/Rule ⅚
2 Loma Linda ¹¹/₁₂
3 McCall ¹⁷/₁₈

Practice Note ▶ Universal Curettes are used on hygiene, periodontal, and operative tray setups.

Sterilization Notes ▶ Universal Curettes must be precleaned, either, placed in a sterilizing pouch with an internal process indicator, sealed, then sterilized OR wrapped with an internal process indicator inside and secured on the outside with process indicator tape, then sterilized. Verify appropriate color change has been achieved in external process indicator immediately after removal from sterilizer then check internal process indicator before treatment. Refer to state regulations for any additional state requirements.

▪INSTRUMENT   Langer Universal Curettes

Functions ▶
To scale supragingival and subgingival surfaces
To remove deposits and stains from teeth
To remove soft tissue lining of periodontal pocket and root planing

Characteristics ▶
Blade—Two cutting edges, with face at 90-degree angle to lower shank
Design function with three bends in the shank, improving posterior access
Langer universal curettes designed with the shank design of a Gracey combined with a universal blade
Single or double ended
Range of sizes

Practice Note ▶
Langer Universal Curettes are used on hygiene and periodontal tray setups.

Sterilization Notes ▶
Langer Universal Curettes must be precleaned, either, placed in a sterilizing pouch with an internal process indicator, sealed, then sterilized OR wrapped with an internal process indicator inside and secured on the outside with process indicator tape, then sterilized. Verify appropriate color change has been achieved in external process indicator immediately after removal from sterilizer then check internal process indicator before treatment. Refer to state regulations for any additional state requirements.

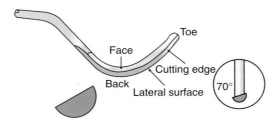

Toe

Face

Cutting edge

Back

Lateral surface

70°

Area-Specific Curettes—Anterior

Functions ▶ To scale and remove deposits from subgingival surfaces of anterior teeth

To use for root planing, periodontal débridement, and soft tissue curettage

Characteristics ▶ Two cutting edges (only lower cutting edge used)

Blade—Rounded back and toe; at 70-degree angle to lower shank; types: standard, rigid, extra rigid

Curvature of blade designed to adapt to specific teeth and surfaces

Range of sizes available: ½, ¾, ⅚

Curette named by designer: Gracey, Kramer-Nevins, Turgeon

Practice Note ▶ Area-specific Curettes—Anterior are used on hygiene and periodontal tray setups.

Sterilization Notes ▶ Area-Specific Curettes must be precleaned, either, placed in a sterilizing pouch with an internal process indicator, sealed, then sterilized OR wrapped with an internal process indicator inside and secured on the outside with process indicator tape, then sterilized. Verify appropriate color change has been achieved in external process indicator immediately after removal from sterilizer then check internal process indicator before treatment. Refer to state regulations for any additional state requirements.

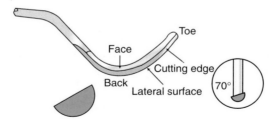

Toe

Face

Cutting edge

Back

Lateral surface

70°

Functions ▶ To scale and remove deposits from subgingival surfaces of posterior teeth

To use for root planing, periodontal deébridement, and soft tissue curettage

Characteristics ▶ Two cutting edges (only lower cutting edge used)

Blade—Rounded back and toe; at 70-degree angle to lower shank; types: standard, rigid, extra rigid

Curvature of blade designed to adapt to specific teeth and surfaces

Range of size, shape, and bends in shank

Two bends in shank

Examples: $7/8$, $9/10$

Three bends in shank

Examples: $11/12$, $13/14$, $15/16$, $17/18$

Curette named by designer: Gracey, Kramer-Nevins, Turgeon

Practice Note ▶ Area-specific Curettes—Posterior are used on hygiene and periodontal tray setups.

Sterilization Notes ▶ Area-specific Curettes must be precleaned, either, placed in a sterilizing pouch with an internal process indicator, sealed, then sterilized OR wrapped with an internal process indicator inside and secured on the outside with process indicator tape, then sterilized. Verify appropriate color change has been achieved in external process indicator immediately after removal from sterilizer then check internal process indicator before treatment. Refer to state regulations for any additional state requirements.

Extended Area-Specific Curettes—Anterior

Function ▶ To scale and remove deposits in deep periodontal pockets 5 mm or deeper

Characteristics ▶ Two cutting edges (only lower cutting edge used)
Blade at 70-degree angle to lower shank; types: standard, rigid, extra rigid
Curvature of blade designed to adapt to anteriors
Terminal shank redesigned—3 mm longer than standard area-specific curette
Manufacturer's trademark name usually follows ½, ¾, ⅚ numbering system
Range of sizes—Commonly used types: ¾, ⅚
Double-ended curettes packaged in sets
Curettes named by designer: Gracey ½

Practice Note ▶ Extended Area-Specific Curettes—Anterior are used on hygiene and periodontal tray setups.

Sterilization Notes ▶ Extended Area-Specific Curettes must be precleaned, either, placed in a sterilizing pouch with an internal process indicator, sealed, then sterilized OR wrapped with an internal process indicator inside and secured on the outside with process indicator tape, then sterilized. Verify appropriate color change has been achieved in external process indicator immediately after removal from sterilizer then check internal process indicator before treatment. Refer to state regulations for any additional state requirements.

Extended Area-Specific Curettes—Posterior

Function ▶ To scale and remove deposits in deep periodontal pockets (5 mm or deeper)

Characteristics ▶ Two cutting edges (only lower cutting edge used)
Blade at 70-degree angle to lower shank; types: standard, rigid, extra rigid
Curvature of blade designed to adapt to premolars, molars
Terminal shank redesigned—3 mm longer than standard area-specific curette
Range of sizes
Commonly used types: $11/12$, $13/14$, $15/16$, $17/18$
Double-ended curettes packaged in sets
Curettes named by designer: Gracey $11/12$ rigid, Gracey $11/12$

Practice Note ▶ Extended Area-Specific Curettes—Posterior are used on hygiene and periodontal tray setups.

Sterilization Notes ▶ Extended Area-Specific Curettes must be precleaned, either, placed in a sterilizing pouch with an internal process indicator, sealed, then sterilized OR wrapped with an internal process indicator inside and secured on the outside with process indicator tape, then sterilized. Verify appropriate color change has been achieved in external process indicator immediately after removal from sterilizer then check internal process indicator before treatment. Refer to state regulations for any additional state requirements.

Mini Extended Area-Specific Curettes—Anterior

Function ▶ To scale in deep periodontal pockets (5 mm)

Characteristics ▶ Blade redesigned to be half the length of extended area-specific curette
Designed for narrow roots, pockets, or furcations
Two cutting edges (only lower cutting edge used)
Blade at 70-degree angle to lower shank; types: standard, rigid, extra rigid
Curvature of blade designed to adapt to anteriors
Range of sizes
Manufacturer's trademark name usually follows ½, ¾, ⅝ numbering system
Curettes named by designer: Gracey ½

Practice Note ▶ Mini Extended Area-Specific Curettes—Anterior are used on hygiene and periodontal tray setups.

Sterilization Notes ▶ Mini Extended Area-Specific Curettes must be precleaned, either, placed in a sterilizing pouch with an internal process indicator, sealed, then sterilized OR wrapped with an internal process indicator inside and secured on the outside with process indicator tape, then sterilized. Verify appropriate color change has been achieved in external process indicator immediately after removal from sterilizer then check internal process indicator before treatment. Refer to state regulations for any additional state requirements.

Mini Extended Area-Specific Curettes—Posterior

Function ▶ To scale in deep periodontal pockets (5 mm)

Characteristics ▶ Blade redesigned to be half the length of extended area-specific curette

Designed for narrow roots, pockets, or furcations

Two cutting edges (only lower cutting edge used)

Blade at 70-degree angle to lower shank; types: standard, rigid, extra rigid

Curvature of blade designed to adapt to premolars, molars

Range of size, shape, and bends in shank available

Two bends in shank

Examples: $\frac{7}{8}$, $\frac{9}{10}$

Three bends in shank

Examples: $\frac{11}{12}$, $\frac{13}{14}$, $\frac{15}{16}$, $\frac{17}{18}$

Curettes named by designer: Gracey $\frac{11}{12}$ mini extender

Practice Note ▶ Mini Extended Area-Specific Curettes—Posterior are used on hygiene and periodontal tray setups.

Sterilization Notes ▶ Mini Extended Area-Specific Curettes must be precleaned, either, placed in a sterilizing pouch with an internal process indicator, sealed, then sterilized OR wrapped with an internal process indicator inside and secured on the outside with process indicator tape, then sterilized. Verify appropriate color change has been achieved in external process indicator immediately after removal from sterilizer then check internal process indicator before treatment. Refer to state regulations for any additional state requirements.

Implant Scaler

Function ▶ To remove deposits and stains from surface of implant

Characteristics ▶
1. Disposable tips (each tip should be sterilized before use). Instrument with disposable tip attached.
2. Titanium-coated scaler

Different designs allow scaling without scratching of titanium implants

Some tips are made of Plasteel—a high-grade resin

Practice Note ▶ Implant Scalers are used on hygiene and periodontal tray setups.

Sterilization Notes ▶ Handle and titanium-coated Scaler must be precleaned, either, placed in a sterilizing pouch with an internal process indicator, sealed, then sterilized OR wrapped with an internal process indicator inside and secured on the outside with process indicator tape, then sterilized. Verify appropriate color change has been achieved in external process indicator immediately after removal from sterilizer then check internal process indicator before treatment. Refer to state regulations for any additional state requirements. Or disposable scaler tip should be disposed of in a sharps container.

Cutting edge

Face

Tip

Cutting edge

Back

Lateral surface

90°

■INSTRUMENT Straight Sickle Scaler

Function ▶ To remove large amounts of deposits from supragingival surfaces

Characteristics ▶ Two cutting edges on straight blade that ends in sharp point
Long; two bends in shank
Variety of sizes and angles
Single or double ended—Two ends may be shaped differently

Practice Note ▶ Straight Sickle Scaler is used on hygiene and periodontal tray setups.

Sterilization Notes ▶ Straight Sickle Scaler must be precleaned, either, placed in a sterilizing pouch with an internal process indicator, sealed, then sterilized OR wrapped with an internal process indicator inside and secured on the outside with process indicator tape, then sterilized. Verify appropriate color change has been achieved in external process indicator immediately after removal from sterilizer then check internal process indicator before treatment. Refer to state regulations for any additional state requirements. Refer to state regulations for any additional state requirements.

1 →

MONTANA JACK® R138
USA CE F106

2 →

svensedge
SH6/79°
Made in USA CE 05

Cutting edge
Tip Face
90°
Cutting edge Back
Lateral surface

Curved Sickle Scaler

Function ▶ To remove large amounts of deposits from supragingival surfaces

Characteristics ▶ Two cutting edges on curved blade that ends in sharp point
Long, straight shank with one gentle bend
Variety of sizes and angles
Single or double ended—Two ends may be shaped differently

1 Montana Jack—Sharper, thinner blades with solid resin handle for comfortable grip.
2 Traditional Curved Sickle Scaler

Practice Note ▶ Curved Sickle Scaler is used on hygiene and periodontal tray setups.

Sterilization Notes ▶ Curved Sickle Scaler must be precleaned, either, placed in a sterilizing pouch with an internal process indicator, sealed, then sterilized OR wrapped with an internal process indicator inside and secured on the outside with process indicator tape, then sterilized. Verify appropriate color change has been achieved in external process indicator immediately after removal from sterilizer then check internal process indicator before treatment. Refer to state regulations for any additional state requirements.

Micro Mini-Five Area-Specific Curette

Function ▶ To scale into periodontal pockets and root surfaces of 5 mm or more

Characteristics ▶ Blade half the length of After Five or standard Gracey curettes
Shank slightly increased rigidity compared with traditional mini five Gracey curettes

Practice Notes ▶ Designed for narrow pockets and furcations
Micro Mini-Five Area-Specific Curette—used on hygiene and periodontal tray setups

Sterilization Notes ▶ Micro Mini-Five Area-Specific Curette must be precleaned, either, placed in a sterilizing pouch with an internal process indicator, sealed, then sterilized OR wrapped with an internal process indicator inside and secured on the outside with process indicator tape, then sterilized. Verify appropriate color change has been achieved in external process indicator immediately after removal from sterilizer then check internal process indicator before treatment. Refer to state regulations for any additional state requirements.

▪INSTRUMENT Magnetostrictive Power Scaler

Function ▶ To use with water-cooled ultrasonic inserts vibrating at high frequency

Characteristics ▶ Ultra-high frequency sound waves convert mechanical energy into vibrations (frequency ranges from 18 to 50 kHz).

Some units (depending on manufacturer) have self-contained water reservoirs.

Some units (depending on manufacturer) have an additional air/water/sodium bicarbonate slurry polishing system to remove extrinsic stains and dental plaque.

A variety of sizes and designs are available.

Practice Note ▶ Magnetostrictive Power Scaler/ Ultrasonic Scaling Unit is used during a routine prophylaxis appointment or for other appointments for root planing.

Sterilization Notes ▶ Barriers should be used for Power Scaler unit. Refer to the manufacturer's recommendation for disinfecting the unit.

Power scaler inserts must be precleaned, either, placed in a sterilizing pouch with an internal process indicator, sealed, then sterilized OR wrapped with an internal process indicator inside and secured on the outside with process indicator tape, then sterilized. Verify appropriate color change has been achieved in external process indicator immediately after removal from sterilizer then check internal process indicator before treatment. Refer to state regulations for any additional state requirements.

Ultrasonic Scaler Instrument Tip—Supragingival

Functions ▶ To remove supragingival calculus from teeth
To remove bacterial plaque from periodontal pockets
To remove heavy debris and stains from teeth
To remove excess cement from orthodontic bands after cementation and after band removal

Characteristics ▶ Supragingival Tip is inserted into the tubing on the ultrasonic scaling unit
Available in different lengths (called stacks): 25 kHz or 30 kHz, depending on unit
Water-cooled inserts (Water systems vary with internal or external water delivery.)
Variety of shapes, sizes, and designs, depending on designated and varying grips
Example: Original prophy
Tip style: Finely beveled internal water delivery tube

Practice Notes ▶ Ultrasonic Scaler Tip—Supragingival is used on hygiene and periodontal tray setups.
These tips are also known as ultrasonic inserts.

Sterilization Notes ▶ Ultrasonic Scaler Tip—Supragingival must be precleaned, either, placed in a sterilizing
pouch with an internal process indicator, sealed, then sterilized OR wrapped with an
internal process indicator inside and secured on the outside with process indicator tape, then
sterilized. Verify appropriate color change has been achieved in external process indicator
immediately after removal from sterilizer then check internal process indicator before
treatment. Refer to state regulations for any additional state requirements.

Ultrasonic Scaler Instrument Tip—Subgingival

Functions ▶ To remove subgingival calculus from teeth
To remove bacterial plaque from periodontal pockets

Characteristics ▶ Subgingival Scaler Tip— is inserted into the tubing on the ultrasonic scaling unit.
Available in different lengths (called stacks): 25 kHz or 30 kHz, depending on unit
Water-cooled inserts (Water systems vary with internal or external water delivery.)
Variety of shapes, sizes, and designs, depending on designated area and varying grips
Example: After Five design
Tip style: Finely beveled internal water delivery tube (pictured)

Practice Notes ▶ Ultrasonic Scaler Tip—Subgingival is used on hygiene and periodontal tray setups.
These tips are also known as ultrasonic inserts.

Sterilization Notes ▶ Ultrasonic Scaler Tip—Subgingival must be precleaned, either, placed in a sterilizing pouch
with an internal process indicator, sealed, then sterilized OR wrapped with an internal
process indicator inside and secured on the outside with process indicator tape, then
sterilized. Verify appropriate color change has been achieved in external process indicator
immediately after removal from sterilizer then check internal process indicator before
treatment. Refer to state regulations for any additional state requirements.

Ultrasonic Scaler Instrument Tip—Furcation

Function ▶ To remove bacterial plaque from furcation areas

Characteristics ▶ Furcation Tip is inserted into the tubing on the ultrasonic scaling unit.
Available in different lengths (called stacks): 25 kHz or 30 kHz, depending on unit
Water-cooled inserts (Water systems vary with internal or external water delivery.)
Variety of shapes, sizes, and designs, depending on designated area and varying grips
Example: Furcation Plus design
Tip style: 0.8-mm ball end adapts to furcation, external water delivery tube (pictured)

Practice Notes ▶ Ultrasonic Scaler Tip—furcation is used on hygiene and periodontal tray setups.
These tips are also known as ultrasonic inserts.
Pictured: Original Prophy

Sterilization Notes ▶ Ultrasonic Scaler Tip—Furcation must be precleaned, either, placed in a sterilizing pouch
with an internal process indicator, sealed, then sterilized OR wrapped with an internal
process indicator inside and secured on the outside with process indicator tape, then
sterilized. Verify appropriate color change has been achieved in external process indicator
immediately after removal from sterilizer then check internal process indicator before
treatment. Refer to state regulations for any additional state requirements.

Ultrasonic Scaler Instrument Tip—Universal

Function ▶ To remove bacterial plaque and general deposits

Characteristics ▶ Universal tip is inserted into the tubing on the ultrasonic scaling unit.
Available in different lengths (called stacks): 25 kHz or 30 kHz, depending on unit
Water-cooled inserts (Water systems vary with internal or external water delivery.)
Variety of shapes, sizes, and designs, depending on designated area and varying grips
Example: Streamline design
Tip style: Water delivered directly from base of tip, eliminating need for external water system; efficient at low settings (pictured)

Practice Notes ▶ Ultrasonic Scaler Tip—universal is used on hygiene and periodontal tray setups.
These tips are also known as ultrasonic inserts.

Sterilization Notes ▶ Ultrasonic Scaler Tip—Universal must be precleaned, either, placed in a sterilizing pouch with an internal process indicator, sealed, then sterilized OR wrapped with an internal process indicator inside and secured on the outside with process indicator tape, then sterilized. Verify appropriate color change has been achieved in external process indicator immediately after removal from sterilizer then check internal process indicator before treatment. Refer to state regulations for any additional state requirements.

Sharpening Stones

Function ▶ To sharpen scalers and curettes

Characteristics ▶ Types of stones:

1 India stones—Remove the most metal when used and should be followed with an Arkansas or ceramic stone

2 Arkansas stones—Provide a polished edge (flat and cone-shaped pictured)

3 Ceramic stones—Provide a polished edge and do not require lubrication

Practice Note ▶ Sharpening Stones are used on hygiene and periodontal tray setups.

Sterilization Notes ▶ Sharpening Stones must be precleaned, either, placed in a sterilizing pouch with an internal process indicator, sealed, then sterilized OR wrapped with an internal process indicator inside and secured on the outside with process indicator tape, then sterilized. Verify appropriate color change has been achieved in external process indicator immediately after removal from sterilizer then check internal process indicator before treatment. Refer to state regulations for any additional state requirements.

Battery-Operated Sharpening Device

Function ▶ To sharpen scalers and curettes

Characteristics ▶ Stone moves underneath a stainless-steel guideplate, which puts the blade at factory angles. Sharpener has a power device with instrument guide channels and a vertical backstop to help control blade angulation. (Pictured: Sidekick Sharpener)

Practice Note ▶ Battery-Operated Sharpening Device should be used with sterile scalers and curettes, and then instruments resterilized after sharpening.

Sterilization Notes ▶ Barrier wrap; disinfect or sterilize certain parts of equipment according to the manufacturer's recommendation. Sterilized instruments must be precleaned, either, placed in a sterilizing pouch with an internal process indicator, sealed, then sterilized OR wrapped with an internal process indicator inside and secured on the outside with process indicator tape, then sterilized. Verify appropriate color change has been achieved in external process indicator immediately after removal from sterilizer then check internal process indicator before treatment. Refer to state regulations for any additional state requirements.

Hygiene

FROM LEFT TO RIGHT

Mouth mirror, explorer, periodontal probe, cotton forceps, curved sickle scaler, 4L/4R universal posterior, universal Langer ½, Ratcliff ¾, Gracey ⅞, Gracey ¹¹/₁₂, Gracey ¹³/₁₄, air/water syringe tip, low-volume saliva ejector, high-volume evacuation (HVE) tip

Sterilization Notes ▶ Refer to each picture for correct procedure for instrument sterilization or disposal of instrument or material. Refer to other chapters for additional instruments on this tray setup that are not included in this chapter.

Root Planing

FROM LEFT TO RIGHT

Mouth mirror, explorer, periodontal probe, cotton forceps, Gracey ½, Gracey ¾, Gracey ⅞, Gracey ¹¹/₁₂, Gracey ¹³/₁₄, air/water syringe tip, low-volume saliva ejector, high-volume evacuation (HVE) tip

Sterilization Notes ▶ Refer to each individual picture for correct procedure for instrument sterilization or disposal of instrument or material. Refer to other chapters for additional instruments on this tray setup that are not included in this chapter.

Preventive and Sealant Instruments and Whitening Trays

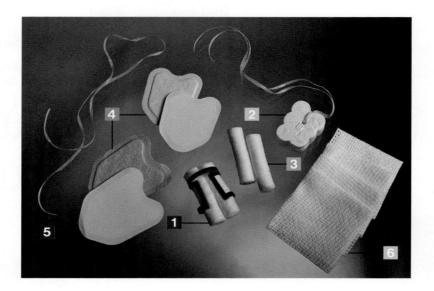

▪INSTRUMENT Disposables

Functions ▶ To use with all types of dental procedures
To use when area in the mouth needs to stay dry

Characteristics ▶

1 Cotton Roll Holder for mandibular arch; one cotton roll is placed on the buccal side of the teeth, and the other is placed on the lingual side of the teeth.

2 Disposable Bite Block with ligature tie for safety as to retrieve if patient swallows bite block.

3 Cotton Rolls

4 Dry Aids for keeping mouth dry—small and large

5 Dental floss

6 2 × 2 gauze

Dry Aid is placed on the buccal mucosa—inside the cheek—opposite the maxillary second molar near the Stensen's duct to absorb saliva originating from the parotid gland.

Practice Note ▶ Disposables are used on all dental tray procedures, including sealant and other restorative tray setups.

Sterilization Notes ▶ All Disposables should be disposed of in the garbage. Single use only.

Fluoride Trays—Disposable

Functions ▶ To fill trays with fluoride; remineralizing enamel
To help prevent decay by mineralizing the teeth

Characteristic ▶ Variety of disposable trays and fluoride available

Practice Note ▶ Fluoride treatment is usually given to children at their
6-month checkup appointment.
Fluoride Trays are used on fluoride tray setups.

Sterilization Notes ▶ Fluoride Trays should be disposed of in the garbage. Single
use only.

Vacuum Former

Functions ▶ To make whitening trays, custom temporary crowns, night guards, orthodontic positioners, and mouth guards
To heat plastic square for bleaching trays
To vacuum form the plastic tray over the patient's model to make the bleaching tray and devices as mentioned above

Characteristics ▶ Heating element that softens the thermoplastic resin
2 Handles to pull down plastic
3 Vacuum to mold plastic to tray after it is pulled down

Practice Note ▶ Block-out material is light cured on the facial side of the model before whitening trays are made with the vacuum former.

Sterilization Notes ▶ The manufacturer's recommendation should be followed for disinfecting the Vacuum Former.

Custom-Fitted Whitening Tray

Function ▶ To lighten the color of dark or discolored teeth

Characteristics ▶ **1** Custom-fitted trays are made in the dental office with the vacuum former.
2 Trays hold a peroxide-based gel.
Different percentages of gel available
Usage regimens vary according to dentist recommendations

Practice Note ▶ Bleaching Trays should stop short of the gingival margin of the soft tissues to avoid gingival irritation.

Sterilization Notes ▶ Clean and disinfect according to dentist's recommendation.

Scissors—Short Blade

Function ▶ To precisely cut material especially for whitening trays.

Characteristic ▶ Fine cutting blade

Practice Note ▶ Short-Blade Scissors are used on whitening tray setup and on other operative tray setups.

Sterilization Notes ▶ Scissors—Short Blade must be precleaned open and unlocked, placed in an open and unlocked position either in a sterilizing pouch with an internal process indicator, sealed, then sterilized OR wrapped with an internal process indicator inside and secured on the outside with process indicator tape, then sterilized. Verify appropriate color change has been achieved in external process indicator immediately after removal from sterilizer then check internal process indicator before treatment. Refer to state regulations for any additional state requirements.

DIAGNOdent

Functions ▶ To aid in the detection of caries within the tooth structure
To detect caries in the structure of the tooth before placing sealants

Characteristics ▶ DIAGNOdent accurately diagnoses occlusal caries.
Laser detects the caries in the tooth, and a digital display is seen on the screen.

Practice Note ▶ DIAGNOdent is used with sealant and occasionally restorative tray setups.

Sterilization Notes ▶ The manufacturer's recommendation should be followed for disinfecting DIAGNOdent unit. Barriers should be placed on wand that is used intraorally. Refer to manufacturer's recommendation for precleaning and sterilization of the DIAGNOdent tips.

Spectra Fluorescence Caries Detection Aid System

Functions ▶ To aid in the detection of caries

To aid in the detection of caries during the restorative phase to verify that all caries have been removed.

Characteristics ▶ Components

- Lightweight handpiece with high resolution, auto-exposure CCD sensor
- Spacer that maintains an appropriate distance between the lens tip and the tooth surface and blocks stray light during examinations
- Cable to connect handpiece to computer

Uses fluorescence to detect caries in fissures and smooth surfaces

Doppler radar-like images provide both color and numerical indicators; in active mode, carious regions appear red, and healthy enamel appears green

120-degree button ring allows the user to freeze, unfreeze, and capture images with one finger.

Practice Note ▶ The Spectra detects decay hidden between the margins of existing composite and amalgam restorations.

Sterilization Notes ▶ The manufacturer's recommendation should be followed for disinfecting Spectra. Barriers should be placed on camera handpiece that is used intraorally. Spacers are reusable however must be precleaned and sterilized before use.

Prophylaxis Polishing

TOP (LEFT TO RIGHT)

Mouth mirror, explorer, cotton forceps, air/water syringe tip, polishing agent without fluoride, dental floss, low-volume saliva ejector, high-volume evacuator (HVE) tip

BOTTOM (LEFT TO RIGHT)

Prophy slow-speed handpiece with disposable prophy angle attachment with polishing cup, disposable prophy angle attachment with tapered brush

Sterilization Notes ▶ Refer to each picture for correct procedure for instrument sterilization or disposal of instrument or material. Refer to other chapters for additional instruments on this tray setup that are not included in this chapter.

Sealant

VERY TOP OF TRAY
Syringe with etchant

TOP ROW (LEFT TO RIGHT)
High-volume evacuator tip (HVE), mouth mirror, explorer, cotton forceps, microbrushes, disposable articulating paper holder and articulating paper, air/water syringe tip, dry aids, low-volume evacuator for mandibular, cotton rolls in disposable holder

BOTTOM ROW (LEFT TO RIGHT)
Disposable bite block, dental floss, sealant syringe and syringe tip, prophy slow-speed hand-piece with disposable prophy angle attachment with polishing cup, disposable prophy angle attachment with tapered brush

Sterilization Notes ▶ Refer to each picture for correct procedure for instrument sterilization or disposal of instrument or material. Refer to other chapters for additional instruments on this tray setup that are not included in this chapter.

Whitening

LEFT TO RIGHT

Thermoplastic resin square, bleaching trays (maxillary and mandibular), short-blade scissors, block-out material for models, bleaching trays on maxillary and mandibular models

Sterilization Notes ▶ Refer to each picture for correct procedure for instrument sterilization or disposal of instrument or material. Refer to other chapters for additional instruments on this tray setup that are not included in this chapter.

Orthodontic Instruments

Elastic Separators

Functions ▶ To separate teeth before banding a tooth for orthodontic treatment
To place around contact area of tooth

Characteristic ▶ Elastomeric separators—Various sizes for different contact areas

Practice Note ▶ Separators are placed on orthodontic separating tray setup.

Sterilization Notes ▶ Elastomeric Separators should be disposed of in the garbage. Single use only.

Elastic Separating Pliers

Function ▶ To grip and place separators around contact area of tooth

Characteristic ▶ Single ended

Practice Note ▶ Elastic Separating Pliers are only used on the orthodontic tray setup.

Sterilization Notes ▶ Elastic Separating Pliers must be precleaned open and unlocked, placed in an open and unlocked position either in a sterilizing pouch with an internal process indicator, sealed, then sterilized OR wrapped with an internal process indicator inside and secured on the outside with process indicator tape, then sterilized. Verify appropriate color change has been achieved in external process indicator immediately after removal from sterilizer then check internal process indicator before treatment. Refer to state regulations for any additional state requirements.

Steel Spring Separators/Brass Wire Separators

Functions ▶ To separate teeth before banding a tooth for orthodontic treatment

To place around contact area of tooth

Characteristics ▶ **1** Steel Spring Separators—Various sizes for different-sized contact areas

2 Brass Wire Separators—Placed around contact and twisted clockwise and then cut 3 mm and tucked in order not to impinge on tissue or occlusion

Placed with orthodontic hemostat or bird beak pliers

Practice Note ▶ Separators are placed on orthodontic separating tray setup.

Sterilization Notes ▶ Steel Spring Separators and Brass Wire Separators should be disposed of in a sharps container. Single use only.

Orthodontic Band with Tubing and Hook

Functions ▸ To fit and cement or bond band around the middle third of the coronal part of the tooth

To hold orthodontic arch wire in place (arch wire moves the teeth, many different shapes and sizes)

To secure headgear in tubing on band

Characteristics ▸
1. Band
2. Tubing:
   Arch wire tube (top)—Holds arch wire in place
   Headgear tube (bottom)—Holds headgear in place
3. Hook—Place where elastics are attached.
   Example: Class II, Class III pull

Practice Note ▸ Orthodontic Band is used on orthodontic banding tray setup.

Sterilization Notes ▸ Orthodontic Band should be disposed of in a sharps container. Single use only.

Band Pusher

Function ▶ To push orthodontic bands into place during try-in and cementing phases

Characteristic ▶ Single or double ended

Practice Note ▶ Band Pusher is only used on the orthodontic tray setup.

Sterilization Notes ▶ Band Pusher must be precleaned, either, placed in a sterilizing pouch with an internal process indicator, sealed, then sterilized OR wrapped with an internal process indicator inside and secured on the outside with process indicator tape, then sterilized. Verify appropriate color change has been achieved in external process indicator immediately after removal from sterilizer then check internal process indicator before treatment. Refer to state regulations for any additional state requirements.

Band Pusher or Plugger with Scaler

Functions ▶ To seat or place orthodontic bands during try-in and cementing phases
To remove excess material after cementation or bonding of bands

Characteristics ▶ Double ended:

1 Band Pusher or Plugger
2 Scaler

Practice Note ▶ Band pusher with scaler is used on the orthodontic tray setup.

Sterilization Notes ▶ Band Pusher or Plugger with Scaler must be precleaned, either, placed in a sterilizing pouch with an internal process indicator, sealed, then sterilized OR wrapped with an internal process indicator inside and secured on the outside with process indicator tape, then sterilized. Verify appropriate color change has been achieved in external process indicator immediately after removal from sterilizer then check internal process indicator before treatment. Refer to state regulations for any additional state requirements.

Band Seater—Bite Stick

Function ▶ To assist seating or placing of orthodontic bands for try-in or cementing phase

Characteristics ▶ Single ended
Available in square tip or triangle tip (pictured)

Practice Notes ▶ The patient bites down on the smooth end of the instrument to apply pressure to seat the band.
Band Seater—Bite Stick is only used on the orthodontic tray setup.

Sterilization Notes ▶ Band Seater—Bite Stick must be precleaned, either, placed in a sterilizing pouch with an internal process indicator, sealed, then sterilized OR wrapped with an internal process indicator inside and secured on the outside with process indicator tape, then sterilized. Verify appropriate color change has been achieved in external process indicator immediately after removal from sterilizer then check internal process indicator before treatment. Refer to state regulations for any additional state requirements.

Orthodontic Bracket

Function ▶ To hold orthodontic arch wire in place (arch wire moves the teeth)

Characteristics ▶ Bracket is bonded to tooth.
Hold arch wire in place
Many different types available:

1 Metal brackets
2 Ceramic brackets (for esthetic purposes)

Practice Note ▶ Orthodontic Brackets are used on orthodontic bonding tray setup.

Sterilization Notes ▶ Orthodontic Brackets should be disposed of in a sharps container. Single use only.

Bracket Placement Card

Function ▶ To place each bracket and/or band on card according to tooth placement in mouth

Characteristic ▶ Tape on card holds brackets in place before they are bonded to teeth.

Practice Note ▶ Bracket Placement Card is only used on the orthodontic tray setup.

Sterilization Notes ▶ Bracket Placement Card should be disposed of in the garbage. Single use only.

Posterior Bracket Placement Pliers

Functions ▶ To hold and carry bracket by placing tip of pliers into slot of bracket
To place bracket on tooth for bonding

Characteristic ▶ Range of sizes

Practice Note ▶ Posterior Bracket Placement Pliers are only used on the orthodontic tray setup.

Sterilization Notes ▶ Posterior Bracket Placement Pliers must be precleaned open and unlocked, placed in an open and unlocked position either in a sterilizing pouch with an internal process indicator, sealed, then sterilized OR wrapped with an internal process indicator inside and secured on the outside with process indicator tape, then sterilized. Verify appropriate color change has been achieved in external process indicator immediately after removal from sterilizer then check internal process indicator before treatment. Refer to state regulations for any additional state requirements.

Anterior Bracket Placement Pliers

Functions ▶ To hold and carry bracket by placing tip of pliers into slot of bracket
To place bracket on tooth for bonding

Characteristic ▶ Range of sizes

Practice Note ▶ Anterior Bracket Placement Pliers are only used on the orthodontic tray setup.

Sterilization Notes ▶ Anterior Bracket Placement Pliers must be precleaned open and unlocked, placed in an open and unlocked position either in a sterilizing pouch with an internal process indicator, sealed, then sterilized OR wrapped with an internal process indicator inside and secured on the outside with process indicator tape, then sterilized. Verify appropriate color change has been achieved in external process indicator immediately after removal from sterilizer then check internal process indicator before treatment. Refer to state regulations for any additional state requirements.

Orthodontic (Shure) Scaler

Functions ▶
To place brackets for bonding (both ends)
To remove separators (scaler end)
To remove elastic ligature ties (scaler end)
To remove excess cement or bonding material
(scaler end)
To check for loose bands and brackets (both ends)

Characteristics ▶
Universal instrument used for several orthodontic
functions
Single ended—Scaler or band pusher
Double ended:

1 Band pusher
2 Orthodontic scaler

Practice Note ▶
Orthodontic Scaler is used on the orthodontic tray setup.

Sterilization Notes ▶
Orthodontic Scaler must be precleaned, either, placed in a sterilizing pouch with an internal
process indicator, sealed, then sterilized OR wrapped with an internal process indicator inside
and secured on the outside with process indicator tape, then sterilized. Verify appropriate
color change has been achieved in external process indicator immediately after removal from
sterilizer then check internal process indicator before treatment. Refer to state
regulations for any additional state requirements.

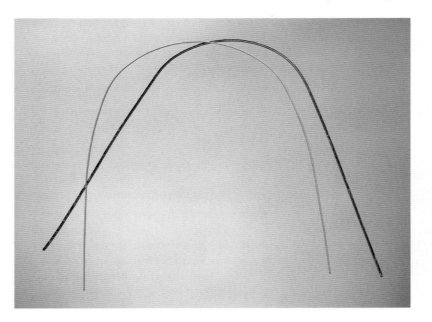

Arch Wire

Function ▶ To place into slots of each bracket and secure with a wire or elastomeric ligature tie on every bracket

To move teeth with the force of the arch wire

Characteristics ▶ Different types of arch wire available according to stage of the orthodontic treatment

Nickel titanium—Flexible wire

Stainless steel wire—Stiff and stronger than other types of wire

Beta titanium—Combination of flexibility, strength, and memory

Optiflex—Made from composite material for light force (initial stages) and esthetic purposes

Different shapes and thickness in diameter available according to initial, intermediate, and advanced treatment:

Round wire—Initial and intermediate stages of treatment

Square, rectangular—Final stages of treatment

Practice Note ▶ Arch Wire is used during all phases of orthodontic treatment when brackets and bands are placed on the teeth.

Sterilization Notes ▶ Arch Wire must be disposed of in a sharps container.

How (or Howe) Pliers

Functions ▶ To place and remove arch wires
To check for loose bands

Characteristics ▶ All-purpose pliers for orthodontic procedures
Serrated tips for better grip on wire
Straight or curved beaks

Practice Note ▶ How Pliers are only used on the orthodontic tray setup.

Sterilization Notes ▶ How Pliers must be precleaned open and unlocked, placed in an open and unlocked position either in a sterilizing pouch with an internal process indicator, sealed, then sterilized OR wrapped with an internal process indicator inside and secured on the outside with process indicator tape, then sterilized. Verify appropriate color change has been achieved in external process indicator immediately after removal from sterilizer then check internal process indicator before treatment. Refer to state regulations for any additional state requirements.

Weingart Utility Pliers

Functions ▶ To place and remove arch wires
To aid a variety of functions for orthodontic procedures
To remove bonded brackets by squeezing bracket

Characteristic ▶ Working ends—Tapered, slim tips to allow pliers to fit between brackets for ease of arch wire placement

Practice Note ▶ Weingart Utility Pliers are only used on the orthodontic tray setup.

Sterilization Notes ▶ Weingart Utility Pliers must be precleaned open and unlocked, placed in an open and unlocked position either in a sterilizing pouch with an internal process indicator, sealed, then sterilized OR wrapped with an internal process indicator inside and secured on the outside with process indicator tape, then sterilized. Verify appropriate color change has been achieved in external process indicator immediately after removal from sterilizer then check internal process indicator before treatment. Refer to state regulations for any additional state requirements.

Arch-Bending Pliers

Function ▶ To bend arch wires

Characteristic ▶ Variety of styles, depending on type of arch wire used—Round, square, or rectangular

Practice Note ▶ Arch-Bending Pliers are only used on the orthodontic tray setup.

Sterilization Notes ▶ Arch-Bending Pliers must be precleaned open and unlocked, placed in an open and unlocked position either in a sterilizing pouch with an internal process indicator, sealed, then sterilized OR wrapped with an internal process indicator inside and secured on the outside with process indicator tape, then sterilized. Verify appropriate color change has been achieved in external process indicator immediately after removal from sterilizer then check internal process indicator before treatment. Refer to state regulations for any additional state requirements.

Tweed Loop-Forming Pliers (Jarabak Pliers)

Functions ▸ To bend and form loops in arch wire
To bend wires for removable appliances

Characteristics ▸ Grooves in beak—Help to bend and form loops in wire
Variety of styles

Practice Note ▸ Tweed Loop-Forming Pliers are only used on the orthodontic tray setup.

Sterilization Notes ▸ Tweed Loop-Forming Pliers must be precleaned open and unlocked, placed in an open and unlocked position either in a sterilizing pouch with an internal process indicator, sealed, then sterilized OR wrapped with an internal process indicator inside and secured on the outside with process indicator tape, then sterilized. Verify appropriate color change has been achieved in external process indicator immediately after removal from sterilizer then check internal process indicator before treatment. Refer to state regulations for any additional state requirements.

Three-Prong Pliers

Function ▶ To contour and bend light wire

Characteristic ▶ Range of sizes available

Practice Note ▶ Three-Prong Pliers are only used on the orthodontic tray setup.

Sterilization Notes ▶ Three-Prong Pliers must be precleaned open and unlocked, placed in an open and unlocked position either in a sterilizing pouch with an internal process indicator, sealed, then sterilized OR wrapped with an internal process indicator inside and secured on the outside with process indicator tape, then sterilized. Verify appropriate color change has been achieved in external process indicator immediately after removal from sterilizer then check internal process indicator before treatment. Refer to state regulations for any additional state requirements.

INSTRUMENT	# Bird Beak Pliers

Functions ▶ To bend and form orthodontic wire
To remove bonded bracket by squeezing bracket

Characteristics ▶ Versatile wire-bending pliers
Beaks on working end meet very precisely

Practice Note ▶ Bird Beak Pliers are only used on the orthodontic tray setup.

Sterilization Notes ▶ Bird Beak Pliers must be precleaned open and unlocked, placed in an open and unlocked position either in a sterilizing pouch with an internal process indicator, sealed, then sterilized OR wrapped with an internal process indicator inside and secured on the outside with process indicator tape, then sterilized. Verify appropriate color change has been achieved in external process indicator immediately after removal from sterilizer then check internal process indicator before treatment. Refer to state regulations for any additional state requirements.

Distal End-Cutting Pliers

Function ▸ To cut distal end of arch wire after placement in brackets and buccal tubes

Characteristic ▸ Catch and hold excess wire after wire has been cut

Practice Note ▸ Distal End-Cutting Pliers are only used on the orthodontic tray setup.

Sterilization Notes ▸ Distal End-Cutting Pliers must be precleaned open and unlocked, placed in an open and unlocked position either in a sterilizing pouch with an internal process indicator, sealed, then sterilized OR wrapped with an internal process indicator inside and secured on the outside with process indicator tape, then sterilized. Verify appropriate color change has been achieved in external process indicator immediately after removal from sterilizer then check internal process indicator before treatment. Refer to state regulations for any additional state requirements.

∎INSTRUMENT Ligatures Ties

Function ▶ To secure the arch wire to the band or bracket

Characteristics ▶
  1 Wire Ligature Ties
  Thin, flexible wire
  Comes in precut length or spools

  2 Kobayashi Ties
  Preformed hook

  3 Elastic Ligature Ties
  Available in different colors
  Comes on a stick (pictured), canes, and chains

Practice Note ▶ Ligature Ties are used on the orthodontic archwire placement tray setup.

Sterilization Notes ▶ Wire Ligature Ties must be disposed of in a sharps container. Elastic ligature ties should be disposed of in garbage.

Ligature-Tying (Coon) Pliers

Function ▶ To tie in ligature to arch wire

Characteristics ▶ Channel on pliers—Locks wire ends in place as tips spread
Variety of styles

Practice Note ▶ Ligature-Tying Pliers are only used on the orthodontic tray setup.

Sterilization Notes ▶ Ligature-Tying Pliers must be precleaned open and unlocked, placed in an open and unlocked position either in a sterilizing pouch with an internal process indicator, sealed, then sterilized OR wrapped with an internal process indicator inside and secured on the outside with process indicator tape, then sterilized. Verify appropriate color change has been achieved in external process indicator immediately after removal from sterilizer then check internal process indicator before treatment. Refer to state regulations for any additional state requirements.

Orthodontic Hemostat

Functions ▶ To hold and place separators
To hold, place, and/or tie ligatures to arch wire

Characteristic ▶ Multifunctional instrument for orthodontic procedures
Example: Mathieu pliers

Practice Note ▶ Orthodontic Hemostat is used on the orthodontic tray setup.

Sterilization Notes ▶ Orthodontic Hemostat must be precleaned open and unlocked, placed in an open and unlocked position either in a sterilizing pouch with an internal process indicator, sealed, then sterilized OR wrapped with an internal process indicator inside and secured on the outside with process indicator tape, then sterilized. Verify appropriate color change has been achieved in external process indicator immediately after removal from sterilizer then check internal process indicator before treatment. Refer to state regulations for any additional state requirements.

Ligature/Wire Cutters

Functions ▶ To cut ligature after it has been tied to arch wire
To cut ligature tie to allow removal of arch wire

Characteristic ▶ Range of sizes available

Practice Note ▶ Ligature/Wire Cutters are used on the orthodontic tray setup.

Sterilization Notes ▶ Ligature/Wire Cutters must be precleaned open and unlocked, placed in an open and unlocked position either in a sterilizing pouch with an internal process indicator, sealed, then sterilized OR wrapped with an internal process indicator inside and secured on the outside with process indicator tape, then sterilized. Verify appropriate color change has been achieved in external process indicator immediately after removal from sterilizer then check internal process indicator before treatment. Refer to state regulations for any additional state requirements.

Ligature Director

Function ▶ To place ligature wire around brackets after it has been tied to arch wire

Characteristics ▶ Single or double ended
Ends of instrument—Have notches to assist placement of ligature tie around brackets

Practice Note ▶ Ligature Director is used on the orthodontic archwire placement tray setup.

Sterilization Notes ▶ Ligature Director must be precleaned, either, placed in a sterilizing pouch with an internal process indicator, sealed, then sterilized OR wrapped with an internal process indicator inside and secured on the outside with process indicator tape, then sterilized. Verify appropriate color change has been achieved in external process indicator immediately after removal from sterilizer then check internal process indicator before treatment. Refer to state regulations for any additional state requirements.

Bracket Placement Card for Damon Self-Ligating Brackets with Self-Ligating Instrument

Functions ► To place each bracket on card according to tooth placement in mouth
Self-Ligating Instrument Instrument—To close bracket around arch wire; ligature tie not needed

Characteristic ► Tape on card holds brackets in place before they are bonded to teeth.

Practice Note ► Bracket Placement Card and self-ligating instrument are used only on orthodontic bonding bracket tray setup.

Sterilization Notes ► Bracket Placement Card should be disposed of in the garbage. Single use only. Self-ligating instrument must be precleaned, either, placed in a sterilizing pouch with an internal process indicator, sealed, then sterilized OR wrapped with an internal process indicator inside and secured on the outside with process indicator tape, then sterilized. Verify appropriate color change has been achieved in external process indicator immediately after removal from sterilizer then check internal process indicator before treatment. Refer to state regulations for any additional state requirements.

Self-Ligating Brackets with Self-Ligating Instrument

Functions ▸ To place each bracket on card according to tooth placement in mouth
Instrument—To open and close bracket around arch wire; ligature tie not needed

Characteristic ▸ Tape on card holds brackets in place before they are bonded to teeth.

Practice Note ▸ Bracket Placement Card and self-ligating instrument are used only on orthodontic bonding
bracket tray setup.

Sterilization Notes ▸ Bracket Placement Card should be disposed of in the garbage. Single use only. Self-ligating
instrument must be precleaned, either, placed in a sterilizing pouch with an internal process
indicator, sealed, then sterilized OR wrapped with an
internal process indicator inside and secured on the
outside with process indicator tape, then sterilized.
Verify appropriate color change has been achieved in
external process indicator immediately after removal
from sterilizer then check internal process indicator
before treatment. Refer to state regulations for any
additional state requirements.

Lip Retractors

Functions ▶ To retract lips, allowing for intraoral access for bonding brackets
To retract lips for intraoral orthodontic photographs

Characteristics ▶ **1** Reusable Lip Retractors
2 Disposable Lip Retractors

Practice Note ▶ Lip Retractors are used with orthodontic procedures and
other tray setups that include taking intraoral photographs.

Sterilization Notes ▶ Reusable Lip Retractors must be precleaned, either, placed
in a sterilizing pouch with an internal process indicator,
sealed, then sterilized OR wrapped with an internal process
indicator inside and secured on the outside with process indicator tape, then sterilized.
Verify appropriate color change has been achieved in external process indicator immediately
after removal from sterilizer then check internal process indicator before treatment. Refer to
state regulations for any additional state requirements. Disposable Lip Retractors should be
disposed of in garbage.

Posterior Band Remover

Function ▶ To remove orthodontic bands from teeth

Characteristics ▶ Two beak types:

1. One beak has round cover to place on occlusal surface of tooth to prevent damage during removal of band. Cover can be replaced.
2. Opposite beak is curved and is placed on gingival side of bracket to apply pressure and remove band from tooth.

Practice Note ▶ Posterior Band Remover is used on the orthodontic tray setup.

Sterilization Notes ▶ Posterior Band Remover must be precleaned open and unlocked, placed in an open and unlocked position either in a sterilizing pouch with an internal process indicator, sealed, then sterilized OR wrapped with an internal process indicator inside and secured on the outside with process indicator tape, then sterilized. Verify appropriate color change has been achieved in external process indicator immediately after removal from sterilizer then check internal process indicator before treatment. Refer to state regulations for any additional state requirements.

Bracket Remover

Function ▶ To remove anterior or posterior brackets from teeth

Characteristic ▶ Grasp bracket to remove it from tooth.

Practice Note ▶ Bracket Remover is used on the orthodontic tray setup.

Sterilization Notes ▶ Bracket Remover must be precleaned open and unlocked, placed in an open and unlocked position either in a sterilizing pouch with an internal process indicator, sealed, then sterilized OR wrapped with an internal process indicator inside and secured on the outside with process indicator tape, then sterilized. Verify appropriate color change has been achieved in external process indicator immediately after removal from sterilizer then check internal process indicator before treatment. Refer to state regulations for any additional state requirements.

Adhesive-Removing Pliers

Function ▶ To remove excess adhesive after debonding of brackets

Characteristics ▶
1 Plastic pad on round end (pad can be changed)
2 Carbide-inserted tip on short beak—Used to remove the bulk of composite material after debonding

Practice Note ▶ Adhesive-Removing Pliers are used on the orthodontic tray setup.

Sterilization Notes ▶ Adhesive-Removing Pliers must be precleaned open and unlocked, placed in an open and unlocked position either in a sterilizing pouch with an internal process indicator, sealed, then sterilized OR wrapped with an internal process indicator inside and secured on the outside with process indicator tape, then sterilized. Verify appropriate color change has been achieved in external process indicator immediately after removal from sterilizer then check internal process indicator before treatment. Refer to state regulations for any additional state requirements.

Invisalign and CEREC Omnicam

Function ▶ To take images with an intraoral Wand/Camera of the maxillary and mandibular arches. Images are sent to the computer.

To send images to a lab to manufacuture Invisalign appliances

Characteristics ▶

1 Wand/Camera that captures images connected to the computer

2 Cerec Omnicam captures the images of teeth in the maxillary and mandibular arches for Invisalign orthodontic appliances that move teeth for Orthodontic procedures.

3 Invisalign appliance

4 Traditional orthodontics

Images are send to the the lab to manufacture a series of Invisalign appliances for Orthodontic movement of the teeth.

Practice Note ▶ The CEREC Omnicam is used mainly for Orthodontic Invisalign appliances

Sterilization Notes ▶ Barriers should be used for the intraoral Wand/Camera. Barriers or overgloves should be used for manipulating the computer on the Cerec Omnicam. Otherwise, refer to the manufacturer's recommendation for disinfecting.

Temporary Anchorage Device (TAD)

Function ▶ To aid in the movement of teeth with skeletal anchorage assisting in orthodontic treatment

Some examples of TAD:

Closure of space between teeth

Tooth uprighting

Open bite correction

To provide an anchor point to move teeth

Characteristics ▶ **1** TAD

2 TAD (arrow) inserted for movement of teeth TADs are small titanium anchors also referred to as mini implants or mini screws. Before placement, chlorhexidine solution (an antibacterial solution) is placed on the area before anesthesia.

TAD surgery procedure is referred by the orthodontist to a periodontist or a maxillofacial surgeon.

Practice Note ▶ TADs are used with periodontal and maxillofacial surgery setups, oral surgery or periodontal surgery setup, and orthodontic tray setups.

Sterilization Notes ▶ TADs must be disposed of in Sharps container. Single use only. Refer to state regulations for any additional state requirements.

Orthodontic Tooth Separating

TOP
Elastic separators, spring coil separators

BOTTOM (LEFT TO RIGHT)
Mouth mirror, explorer, cotton forceps (pliers), orthodontic (Shure) scaler, elastic separating pliers, floss, orthodontic hemostat (Mathieu pliers), air/water syringe tip, low-volume saliva ejector tip, high-volume evacuation (HVE) tip

Sterilization Notes ▶ Refer to each individual picture for correct procedure for instrument sterilization or disposal of instrument or material. Refer to other chapters for additional instruments on this tray setup that are not included in this chapter.

Orthodontic Cementing and Bonding Brackets

TOP ROW (LEFT TO RIGHT)

Bracket placement card with brackets, orthodontic bands, polishing agent without fluoride or glycerin, disposable prophy angle with polishing cup, air/water syringe tip

BOTTOM ROW (LEFT TO RIGHT)

Mouth mirror, explorer, cotton forceps, orthodontic scaler (Shure scaler), band seater-bite stick, posterior band remover, anterior bracket placement pliers, posterior bracket placement pliers, flexible cement spatula, low-volume saliva ejector, high-volume evacuation (HVE) tip, microbrushes, disposable cheek retractors

Sterilization Notes ▶ Refer to each individual picture for correct procedure for instrument sterilization or disposal of instrument or material. Refer to other chapters for additional instruments on this tray setup that are not included in this chapter.

Orthodontic Tying-In Arch Wire

TOP (LEFT TO RIGHT)
Preformed archwire, elastic ligature ties

BOTTOM (LEFT TO RIGHT)
Mouth mirror, explorer, cotton forceps, orthodontic (Shure) scaler, ligature director, wire ligature ties, orthodontic hemostat (Mathieu pliers), (under orthodontic hemostat, short wire ligature ties), ligature-tying (Coon) pliers, bird beak pliers, arch-bending pliers, distal-end cutting pliers, How (Howe) pliers, ligature/wire cutters

Sterilization Notes ▶ Refer to each picture for correct procedure for instrument sterilization or disposal of instrument or material. Refer to other chapters for additional instruments on this tray setup that are not included in this chapter.

Orthodontic Removing Bands and Brackets

LEFT TO RIGHT

Mouth mirror, explorer, cotton forceps, orthodontic (Shure) scaler, posterior band remover, bird beak pliers, universal curette, low-volume saliva ejector, high-volume evacuation (HVE) tip, air/water syringe tip

Sterilization Notes ▶ Refer to each picture for correct procedure for instrument sterilization or disposal of instrument or material. Refer to other chapters for additional instruments on this tray setup that are not included in this chapter.

Universal Surgical Instruments

Mouth Prop

Function ▶ To hold patient's mouth open during dental procedures

Characteristics ▶ Placed in posterior part of mouth while patient bites down
Often used for sedated patients
Disposable mouth props available
Range of sizes—Pediatric to large adult

Practice Notes ▶ Mouth Prop could be used with any dental procedure, including but not exclusive to operative or surgical. Ligate with floss for safety of patient choking.

Sterilization Notes ▶ Mouth Prop must be precleaned, either, placed in a sterilizing pouch with an internal process indicator, sealed, then sterilized OR wrapped with an internal process indicator inside and secured on the outside with process indicator tape, then sterilized. Verify appropriate color change has been achieved in external process indicator immediately after removal from sterilizer then check internal process indicator before treatment. Refer to state regulations for any additional state requirements. Disposable Mouth Props should be disposed of in garbage. Single use only.

Mouth Gag

Function ▶ To hold patient's mouth open during dental procedures

Characteristics ▶ Often used for sedated patients
Locking device
Range of sizes available

Practice Note ▶ Mouth Gag is mostly used for oral surgery and periodontal surgical procedures when patient is sedated.

Sterilization Notes ▶ Mouth Gag must be precleaned open and unlocked, placed in an open and unlocked position either in a sterilizing pouch with an internal process indicator, sealed, then sterilized OR wrapped with an internal process indicator inside and secured on the outside with process indicator tape, then sterilized. Verify appropriate color change has been achieved in external process indicator immediately after removal from sterilizer then check internal process indicator before treatment. Refer to state regulations for any additional state requirements.

Scalpel Handle with Blades

Functions ▶ Handle:
To hold blade in place
Blades:
To cut tissue with blade
To trim interproximal restorations

Characteristics ▶
1 Disposable Handle/Blade in one unit
2 Scalpel Handle

Blades—Disposable, variety of shapes and sizes:

3 #12 Blade
4 #15 Blade

Practice Note ▶ Scalpel with Blades mostly used on oral surgery and periodontal surgical tray
setups and occasionally used with composite tray setups for removing flash material and interproximal carving.

Sterilization Notes ▶ Scalpel Handle must be precleaned, either, placed in a sterilizing pouch with an internal process indicator,
sealed, then sterilized OR wrapped with an internal process indicator inside and secured on the outside with
process indicator tape, then sterilized. Verify appropriate color change has been achieved in external process
indicator immediately after removal from sterilizer then check internal process indicator before treatment.
Refer to state regulations for any additional state requirements. Scalpel blade must be disposed of in a sharps
container. Disposable handle and blade in one unit must be disposed of in a sharps container.

∎INSTRUMENT Scalpel Blade Remover

Function ▶ To safely remove blade from scalpel handle

Characteristics ▶ Removes all sizes of blades
Autoclavable

Practice Notes ▶ Steps for removing blade:

1 Insert blade with blade side up; align to notch.

2 Press down on blade remover.

3 Pull handle away from blade.

Scalpel Blade Remover is mostly used on oral surgery and periodontal surgical tray setups.

Sterilization Notes ▶ Scalpel Blade Remover must be precleaned, either, placed in a sterilizing pouch with an internal process indicator, sealed, then sterilized OR wrapped with an internal process indicator inside and secured on the outside with process indicator tape, then sterilized. Verify appropriate color change has been achieved in external process indicator immediately after removal from sterilizer then check internal process indicator before treatment. Refer to state regulations for any additional state requirements. Scalpel blade must be disposed of in a sharps container.

Tissue Scissors

Function ▶ To cut tissue

Characteristics ▶ Straight or curved
Variety of shapes and sizes
Variety of uses

Practice Note ▶ Tissue Scissors are mostly used on oral surgery and periodontal surgical tray setups.

Sterilization Notes ▶ Tissue Scissors must be precleaned open and unlocked, placed in an open and unlocked position either in a sterilizing pouch with an internal process indicator, sealed, then sterilized OR wrapped with an internal process indicator inside and secured on the outside with process indicator tape, then sterilized. Verify appropriate color change has been achieved in external process indicator immediately after removal from sterilizer then check internal process indicator before treatment. Refer to state regulations for any additional state requirements.

■INSTRUMENT Tissue Forceps

Function ▶ To hold tissue during surgical procedures

Characteristics ▶ Serrated or rat-tooth tips
Range of sizes available

Practice Note ▶ Tissue Forceps are mostly used on oral surgery and periodontal surgical tray setups.

Sterilization Notes ▶ Tissue Forceps must be precleaned, either, placed in a sterilizing pouch with an internal process indicator, sealed, then sterilized OR wrapped with an internal process indicator inside and secured on the outside with process indicator tape, then sterilized. Verify appropriate color change has been achieved in external process indicator immediately after removal from sterilizer then check internal process indicator before treatment. Refer to state regulations for any additional state requirements.

Hemostat

Function ▶ To grasp tissue or bone fragments
To hold and grasp material in and out of the oral cavity

Characteristics ▶ Straight or curved
Working end—Serrated and/or locking
Variety of functions in other dental procedures
Range of sizes available

Practice Notes ▶ Hemostat is mostly used on oral surgery and periodontal surgical tray setups.
Hemostat is also used on restorative and many other tray setups.

Sterilization Notes ▶ Hemostat must be precleaned open and unlocked, placed in an open and unlocked position either in a sterilizing pouch with an internal process indicator, sealed, then sterilized OR wrapped with an internal process indicator inside and secured on the outside with process indicator tape, then sterilized. Verify appropriate color change has been achieved in external process indicator immediately after removal from sterilizer then check internal process indicator before treatment. Refer to state regulations for any additional state requirements.

Periosteal Elevator

Functions ▶ To separate tissue from tooth or bone
To hold tissue away from surgical site

Characteristics ▶ Working end—Pointed or round
Range of sizes available

Practice Note ▶ Periosteal Elevator is used on oral surgery and periodontal
surgical tray setups.

Sterilization Notes ▶ Periosteal Elevator must be precleaned, either, placed
in a sterilizing pouch with an internal process indicator,
sealed, then sterilized OR wrapped with an internal process
indicator inside and secured on the outside with process
indicator tape, then sterilized. Verify appropriate color change has been achieved in external
process indicator immediately after removal from sterilizer then check internal process
indicator before treatment. Refer to state regulations for any additional state requirements.

Surgical Curette

Functions ▶ To remove debris or granulation tissue from surgical site
To remove cyst from extraction site or surgical site
To perform gross tissue débridement

Characteristics ▶ Single or double ended
Variety of sizes and shapes
Examples of commonly used types:

1 Prichard
2 Miller

Practice Note ▶ Surgical Curette is mostly used on oral surgery and periodontal surgical tray setups.

Sterilization Notes ▶ Surgical Curette must be precleaned, either, placed in a sterilizing pouch with an internal process indicator, sealed, then sterilized OR wrapped with an internal process indicator inside and secured on the outside with process indicator tape, then sterilized. Verify appropriate color change has been achieved in external process indicator immediately after removal from sterilizer then check internal process indicator before treatment. Refer to state regulations for any additional state requirements.

Tongue and Cheek Retractor

Function ▶ To hold and retract tongue or cheek during surgery

Characteristic ▶ Variety of styles and sizes
Example of commonly used type: Minnesota (pictured)

Practice Note ▶ Tongue and Cheek Retractor is mostly used on oral surgery and periodontal surgical tray setups.

Sterilization Notes ▶ Tongue and Cheek Retractor must be precleaned, either, placed in a sterilizing pouch with an internal process indicator, sealed, then sterilized OR wrapped with an internal process indicator inside and secured on the outside with process indicator tape, then sterilized. Verify appropriate color change has been achieved in external process indicator immediately after removal from sterilizer then check internal process indicator before treatment. Refer to state regulations for any additional state requirements.

	Surgical Needle Holder

Function ▶ To grasp and manipulate suture needle during use

Characteristics ▶ Working end—Different lengths, curved or straight

Notched ends available (to accommodate needle)

Range of sizes—Micro for microsurgery to large

Variety of styles:

 Universal

2 Castroviejo

Practice Note ▶ Needle Holder is mostly used on oral surgery and periodontal surgical tray setups.

Sterilization Notes ▶ Needle Holder must be precleaned open and unlocked, placed in an open and unlocked position either in a sterilizing pouch with an internal process indicator, sealed, then sterilized OR wrapped with an internal process indicator inside and secured on the outside with process indicator tape, then sterilized. Verify appropriate color change has been achieved in external process indicator immediately after removal from sterilizer then check internal process indicator before treatment. Refer to state regulations for any additional state requirements.

Suture Needle and Sutures

Function ▶ To suture surgical site

Characteristics ▶ Resorbable sutures—Gut plain, chromic gut, polyglycolic acid (PGA)
Nonresorbable sutures—Silk, nylon, polyester, polypropylene
Available in sterile package
Variety of suture needle sizes available with different sutures

Practice Note ▶ Suture Needle and Sutures are mostly used on oral surgery and periodontal surgical tray setups.

Sterilization Notes ▶ Suture Needle and Sutures must be disposed of in a sharps container.

Suture Scissors

Function ▶ To cut sutures

Characteristics ▶ Cutting edges—Straight or angled
May have notch on end of cutting edge (shown in picture)
Range of sizes

Practice Note ▶ Suture Scissors are mostly used on oral surgery and periodontal surgical tray setups.

Sterilization Notes ▶ Suture Scissors must be precleaned open and unlocked, placed in an open and unlocked position either in a sterilizing pouch with an internal process indicator, sealed, then sterilized OR wrapped with an internal process indicator inside and secured on the outside with process indicator tape, then sterilized. Verify appropriate color change has been achieved in external process indicator immediately after removal from sterilizer then check internal process indicator before treatment. Refer to state regulations for any additional state requirements.

Universal Surgical

TOP ROW (LEFT TO RIGHT)

Mouth mirror, explorer, cotton forceps (pliers), scalpel with #12 blade, periosteal elevator, surgical curette (Prichard), tissue forceps, hemostat, tissue scissors, mouth prop, needle holder, suture scissors, tongue and cheek retractor, disposable high-volume surgical evacuation tip, high-volume surgical evacuation tip

BOTTOM ROW

Silk suture with needle in sterile package

Sterilization Notes ▶ Refer to each picture for correct procedure for instrument sterilization or disposal of instrument or material. Refer to other chapters for additional instruments on this tray setup that are not included in this chapter.

Periodontal Instruments and Periodontal Surgical Instruments

Periodontal Probes

Function ▶ To measure periodontal pocket depth in millimeter increments

Characteristics ▶ Flat or rounded ends

Millimeter-increment markings vary for each style:

1 Color coded—Black markings for millimeter measurements

2 Other styles—Indentations in metal for millimeter measurement-each indentation represents a millimeter.

3 Color-ended probe with black visible markings— Replaceable tip, different tip designs, plastic tip safe for implant probing

Double-ended style available with probe on one end and explorer on the other
Computerized probes available

Practice Note ▶ Periodontal Probe is used on basic setup, dental hygiene, and periodontal tray setups.

Sterilization Notes ▶ Periodontal Probes must be precleaned, either, placed in a sterilizing pouch with an internal process indicator, sealed, then sterilized OR wrapped with an internal process indicator inside and secured on the outside with process indicator tape, then sterilized. Verify appropriate color change has been achieved in external process indicator immediately after removal from sterilizer then check internal process indicator before treatment. Refer to state regulations for any additional state requirements.

Furcation Probe

Function ▶ To measure horizontal and vertical pocket depth of multirooted teeth in furcation areas

Characteristics ▶ Flat or rounded ends
Single or double ended
Millimeter-increment markings vary for each style:
- Color coded—Black markings for millimeter measurements
- Other styles—Indentations in metal for millimeter measurements

Example. Nabors probe (color coded)

Practice Note ▶ Furcation Probe is used on basic, dental hygiene, and periodontal tray setups.

Sterilization Notes ▶ Furcation Probes must be precleaned, placed in sterilization pouch or bag and sealed or wrapped and secured with processing indicating tape, and then sterilized. An internal processing indicator should be included with each sterilization pouch or wrap. When an internal processing indicator is not visible, then an external processing indicator should be placed on the outside of the packaging. Indicators should be checked immediately upon removal from sterilizer to verify the appropriate color change has been achieved. Refer to state regulations for any additional state requirements.

Hoe Scaler—Mesial/Distal and Buccal/Lingual

Function ▶ To remove subgingival and supragingival calculus

Characteristics ▶
1 Mesial/Distal Hoe
2 Buccal/Lingual Hoe scaler
Used with pulling motion
Straight cutting edge
Single or double ended
Designed to function in anterior or posterior locations
- Anterior—Shorter, straighter shanks
- Posterior—Longer, angled shanks

Practice Note ▶ Mesial/Distal and Buccal/Lingual Hoe scalers, according to procedure performed, could be used on dental hygiene and periodontal tray setups.

Sterilization Notes ▶ Mesial/Distal and Buccal/Lingual Hoes scalers must be precleaned, either, placed in a sterilizing pouch with an internal process indicator, sealed, then sterilized OR wrapped with an internal process indicator inside and secured on the outside with process indicator tape, then sterilized. Verify appropriate color change has been achieved in external process indicator immediately after removal from sterilizer then check internal process indicator before treatment. Refer to state regulations for any additional state requirements.

Back-Action Hoe

Function ▶ To remove bone adjacent to teeth without causing trauma

Characteristics ▶ Double ended
Variety of sizes and shapes

Practice Note ▶ Back-Action Hoe, according to procedure performed, could be used on dental hygiene and periodontal tray setups.

Sterilization Notes ▶ Back-Action Hoe must be precleaned, either, placed in a sterilizing pouch with an internal process indicator, sealed, then sterilized OR wrapped with an internal process indicator inside and secured on the outside with process indicator tape, then sterilized. Verify appropriate color change has been achieved in external process indicator immediately after removal from sterilizer then check internal process indicator before treatment. Refer to state regulations for any additional state requirements.

Periodontal Knife—Kidney Shaped

Functions ▶ To use for bevel incision for gingivectomy
To use for gingivoplasty

Characteristics ▶ Variety of sizes and shapes
Named by designer: Kirkland, Goldman-Fox, Buck, Solt

Practice Note ▶ Periodontal Knife—kidney shaped is used on periodontal
surgical tray setups.

Sterilization Notes ▶ Periodontal Knife—Kidney Shaped must be precleaned,
either, placed in a sterilizing pouch with an internal process
indicator, sealed, then sterilized OR wrapped with an
internal process indicator inside and secured on the outside with process indicator tape, then
sterilized. Verify appropriate color change has been achieved in external process indicator
immediately after removal from sterilizer then check internal process indicator before
treatment. Refer to state regulations for any additional state requirements.

Interdental Knife—Spear Point

Functions ▶ To use for interdental cutting of gingiva
To remove tissue

Characteristics ▶ Blade angulated for easier use
Named by designer: Orban, Goldman-Fox, Buck, Sanders
Single or double ended
Range of sizes
Example: Buck ⅚

Practice Note ▶ Interdental Knife—spear point is used on periodontal surgical tray setups.

Sterilization Notes ▶ Interdental Knife—Spear Point must be precleaned, either, placed in a sterilizing pouch
with an internal process indicator, sealed, then sterilized OR wrapped with an internal
process indicator inside and secured on the outside with process indicator tape, then
sterilized. Verify appropriate color change has been achieved in external process indicator
immediately after removal from sterilizer then check internal process indicator before
treatment. Refer to state regulations for any additional state requirements.

▪INSTRUMENT Interdental File

Function ▶ To crush and remove heavy deposits from subgingival and supragingival interproximal areas

Characteristics ▶ Used with push or pull motion

Various angles—Curved, straight, mesial/distal, and buccal/lingual

Examples: Sugarman, Schluger, Buck

Range of sizes available

Practice Note ▶ Interdental File is used on periodontal surgical tray setups.

Sterilization Notes ▶ Interdental File must be precleaned, either, placed in a sterilizing pouch with an internal process indicator, sealed, then sterilized OR wrapped with an internal process indicator inside and secured on the outside with process indicator tape, then sterilized. Verify appropriate color change has been achieved in external process indicator immediately after removal from sterilizer then check internal process indicator before treatment. Refer to state regulations for any additional state requirements.

Periodontal Surgical

TOP ROW—LEFT TO RIGHT

Mouth mirror, explorer, cotton forceps (pliers), periodontal probe, furcation probe, mesial/distal hoe, buccal/lingual hoe, back-action hoe, kidney-shaped periodontal knife, interproximal knife, bone file, tissue forceps, surgical curette, periosteal elevator

BOTTOM ROW—LEFT TO RIGHT

Tissue scissors, scalpel with #12 blade, hemostat, silk sutures with needle, needle holder, suture scissors, cheek and tongue retractor (Minnesota), mouth prop, disposable high-volume surgical evacuation tip

Sterilization Notes ▶ Refer to each picture for correct procedure for instrument sterilization or disposal of instrument or material. Refer to Chapter 15 for complete instruments used in periodontal surgery. Also refer to other chapters for additional instruments on tray setup that are not included in this chapter.

Oral Surgery Extraction Instruments

Straight Elevator

Functions ▶ To loosen tooth from periodontal ligaments before
extraction
To separate and lift tooth from socket

Characteristics ▶ Single ended
Range of sizes available

Practice Note ▶ Straight Elevator is used on surgical extraction tray
setups.

Sterilization Notes ▶ Straight Elevator must be precleaned, either, placed in
a sterilizing pouch with an internal process indicator,
sealed, then sterilized OR wrapped with an internal process indicator inside and secured
on the outside with process indicator tape, then sterilized. Verify appropriate color change
has been achieved in external process indicator immediately after removal from sterilizer
then check internal process indicator before treatment. Refer to state regulations for any
additional state requirements.

Luxating Elevator

Functions ▶ To cut periodontal ligaments before extraction
To rock tooth back and forth before extraction

Characteristics ▶ Single ended
Sharp blade on working end
Blade is serrated
Range of sizes available

Practice Note ▶ Luxating Elevator is used on surgical extraction tray setups.

Sterilization Notes ▶ Luxating Elevator must be precleaned, either, placed in a sterilizing pouch with an internal process indicator, sealed, then sterilized OR wrapped with an internal process indicator inside and secured on the outside with process indicator tape, then sterilized. Verify appropriate color change has been achieved in external process indicator immediately after removal from sterilizer then check internal process indicator before treatment. Refer to state regulations for any additional state requirements.

Periotomes

Functions ▶ To cut periodontal ligaments for atraumatic tooth extraction
To use when dental implant placement is indicated

Characteristics ▶ Thin, sharp blades—Cause minimal damage to periodontal ligaments and surrounding alveolar bone
Straight or angled blades
Single or double ended
Range of sizes available
Some manufacturers make replaceable tip.

Practice Note ▶ Periotomes are used on surgical extraction tray setups.

Sterilization Notes ▶ Periotomes must be precleaned, either, placed in a sterilizing pouch with an internal process indicator, sealed, then sterilized OR wrapped with an internal process indicator inside and secured on the outside with process indicator tape, then sterilized. Verify appropriate color change has been achieved in external process indicator immediately after removal from sterilizer then check internal process indicator before treatment. Refer to state regulations for any additional state requirements.

Root Elevators

Functions ▶ To loosen root
To separate and lift root from socket
To use on posterior teeth

Characteristics ▶ Single ended
Right and left pairs
Range of sizes available
Example: Cryer (commonly used type)

Practice Note ▶ Root Elevators are used in surgical extraction tray setups.

Sterilization Notes ▶ Root Elevators must be precleaned, either, placed in a
sterilizing pouch with an internal process indicator, sealed, then sterilized OR wrapped
with an internal process indicator inside and secured on the outside with process indicator
tape, then sterilized. Verify appropriate color change has been achieved in external process
indicator immediately after removal from sterilizer then check internal process indicator
before treatment. Refer to state regulations for any additional state requirements.

T-Bar Elevators

Functions ▶ To loosen tooth from periodontal ligaments before extraction
To separate tooth from alveolus
To use on posterior teeth

Characteristics ▶ Single ended
Rounded or pointed
Right or left pairs
T-bar Elevators are available with different style handles
Range of sizes available

Practice Note ▶ T-bar Elevators are used on surgical extraction tray setups.

Sterilization Notes ▶ T-bar Elevators must be precleaned, either, placed in a sterilizing pouch with an internal process indicator, sealed, then sterilized OR wrapped with an internal process indicator inside and secured on the outside with process indicator tape, then sterilized. Verify appropriate color change has been achieved in external process indicator immediately after removal from sterilizer then check internal process indicator before treatment. Refer to state regulations for any additional state requirements.

Root-Tip Elevators

Function ▶ To lift and remove fragments of root

Characteristics ▶ Single ended
Rounded or pointed
Working ends are serrated
Straight or right and left pairs

Practice Note ▶ Root-tip Elevators are used on surgical extraction tray setups.

Sterilization Notes ▶ Root-Tip Elevators must be precleaned, either, placed in a sterilizing pouch with an internal process indicator, sealed, then sterilized OR wrapped with an internal process indicator inside and secured on the outside with process indicator tape, then sterilized. Verify appropriate color change has been achieved in external process indicator immediately after removal from sterilizer then check internal process indicator before treatment. Refer to state regulations for any additional state requirements.

Root-Tip Picks

Function ▶ To lift and remove small root tips in difficult areas

Characteristics ▶ Pointed at working end
Straight or right and left pairs

Practice Note ▶ Root-tip Picks are used on surgical extraction tray setups.

Sterilization Notes ▶ Root-Tip Picks must be precleaned, either, placed in a sterilizing pouch with an internal process indicator, sealed, then sterilized OR wrapped with an internal process indicator inside and secured on the outside with process indicator tape, then sterilized. Verify appropriate color change has been achieved in external process indicator immediately after removal from sterilizer then check internal process indicator before treatment. Refer to state regulations for any additional state requirements.

Rongeurs

Functions ▶ To trim and remove excess alveolar bone after extraction of teeth
To contour alveolar bone after single or multiple extractions

Characteristics ▶ Variety of sizes and angles
Beaks have cutting edges

Practice Note ▶ Rongeurs used on surgical extraction tray setups.

Sterilization Notes ▶ Rongeurs must be precleaned open and unlocked, placed in an open and unlocked position either in a sterilizing pouch with an internal process indicator, sealed, then sterilized OR wrapped with an internal process indicator inside and secured on the outside with process indicator tape, then sterilized. Verify appropriate color change has been achieved in external process indicator immediately after removal from sterilizer then check internal process indicator before treatment. Refer to state regulations for any additional state requirements.

Bone File

Function ▶ To remove or smooth rough edges of alveolar bone

Characteristics ▶ Used with push-pull motion
Straight-cut or crosscut cutting end
Variety of sizes, angles, and shapes

Practice Note ▶ Bone File is used on surgical extraction tray setups.

Sterilization Notes ▶ Bone File must be precleaned, either, placed in a sterilizing
pouch with an internal process indicator, sealed, then
sterilized OR wrapped with an internal process indicator
inside and secured on the outside with process indicator tape,
then sterilized. Verify appropriate color change has been
achieved in external process indicator immediately after removal from sterilizer then check
internal process indicator before treatment. Refer to state regulations for any additional state
requirements.

Surgical Chisel

Functions ▶ To split or section a tooth for easier removal by tapping on chisel with mallet
To reshape or contour alveolar bone

Characteristics ▶ Single-bevel chisel—For contouring or removing alveolar bone
Bi-bevel chisel—For splitting teeth
Styles—Surgical chisel, bone splitter
Range of sizes available

Practice Note ▶ Surgical Chisel is used on surgical extraction and other types of surgical procedure tray setups.

Sterilization Notes ▶ Surgical Chisel must be precleaned, either, placed in a sterilizing pouch with an internal process indicator, sealed, then sterilized OR wrapped with an internal process indicator inside and secured on the outside with process indicator tape, then sterilized. Verify appropriate color change has been achieved in external process indicator immediately after removal from sterilizer then check internal process indicator before treatment. Refer to state regulations for any additional state requirements.

■INSTRUMENT Surgical Mallet

Functions ▶ To use with bone chisel to section tooth for easier removal by tapping on chisel with surgical mallet
To use with bone chisel to reshape or contour alveolar bone

Characteristic ▶ Range of sizes available

Practice Note ▶ Surgical Mallet is used on surgical extraction and other types of surgical procedure tray setups.

Sterilization Notes ▶ Surgical Mallet must be precleaned, either, placed in a sterilizing pouch with an internal process indicator, sealed, then sterilized OR wrapped with an internal process indicator inside and secured on the outside with process indicator tape, then sterilized. Verify appropriate color change has been achieved in external process indicator immediately after removal from sterilizer then check internal process indicator before treatment. Refer to state regulations for any additional state requirements.

Universal Maxillary Forceps No. 10S

Function ▶ To extract maxillary molars

Characteristic ▶ Straight handle

Practice Note ▶ Universal Maxillary Forceps No. 10S are used on surgical extraction tray setups.

Sterilization Notes ▶ Universal Maxillary Forceps No. 10S must be precleaned open and unlocked, placed in an open and unlocked position either in a sterilizing pouch with an internal process indicator, sealed, then sterilized OR wrapped with an internal process indicator inside and secured on the outside with process indicator tape, then sterilized. Verify appropriate color change has been achieved in external process indicator immediately after removal from sterilizer then check internal process indicator before treatment. Refer to state regulations for any additional state requirements.

Universal Mandibular Forceps No. 16

Function ▶ To extract mandibular first and second molars

Characteristics ▶ Straight handles or one curved handle
Referred to as cowhorn forceps

Practice Note ▶ Universal Mandibular Forceps No. 16 (cowhorn) are used on surgical extraction tray setups.

Sterilization Notes ▶ Universal Mandibular Forceps No. 16 must be precleaned open and unlocked, placed in an open and unlocked position either in a sterilizing pouch with an internal process indicator, sealed, then sterilized OR wrapped with an internal process indicator inside and secured on the outside with process indicator tape, then sterilized. Verify appropriate color change has been achieved in external process indicator immediately after removal from sterilizer then check internal process indicator before treatment. Refer to state regulations for any additional state requirements.

Mandibular Forceps No. 17

Function ▶ To extract bifurcated mandibular first or second molars

Characteristic ▶ Straight handles

Practice Note ▶ Mandibular Forceps No. 17 are used on surgical extraction tray setups.

Sterilization Notes ▶ Mandibular Forceps No. 17 must be precleaned open and unlocked, placed in an open and unlocked position either in a sterilizing pouch with an internal process indicator, sealed, then sterilized OR wrapped with an internal process indicator inside and secured on the outside with process indicator tape, then sterilized. Verify appropriate color change has been achieved in external process indicator immediately after removal from sterilizer then check internal process indicator before treatment. Refer to state regulations for any additional state requirements.

Maxillary Right Forceps No. 88R

Function ▶ To extract trifurcated maxillary right first or second molars

Characteristic ▶ Right split beak—For engaging lingual root

Practice Note ▶ Maxillary Right Forceps No. 88R are used on surgical extraction tray setups.

Sterilization Notes ▶ Maxillary Right Forceps No. 88R must be precleaned open and unlocked, placed in an open and unlocked position either in a sterilizing pouch with an internal process indicator, sealed, then sterilized OR wrapped with an internal process indicator inside and secured on the outside with process indicator tape, then sterilized. Verify appropriate color change has been achieved in external process indicator immediately after removal from sterilizer then check internal process indicator before treatment. Refer to state regulations for any additional state requirements.

Maxillary Left Forceps No. 88L

Function ▶ To extract trifurcated maxillary left first or second molars

Characteristic ▶ Left split beak—For engaging lingual root

Practice Note ▶ Maxillary Left Forceps No. 88L are used on surgical extraction tray setups.

Sterilization Notes ▶ Maxillary Left Forceps No. 88L must be precleaned open and unlocked, placed in an open and unlocked position either in a sterilizing pouch with an internal process indicator, sealed, then sterilized OR wrapped with an internal process indicator inside and secured on the outside with process indicator tape, then sterilized. Verify appropriate color change has been achieved in external process indicator immediately after removal from sterilizer then check internal process indicator before treatment. Refer to state regulations for any additional state requirements.

Maxillary Universal Forceps—Cryer 150

Function ▶ To extract maxillary centrals, laterals, cuspids, premolars, and roots

Characteristics ▶ Straight handles or one curved handle

Practice Note ▶ Maxillary Universal Forceps—Cryer 150 are used on surgical extraction tray setups.

Sterilization Notes ▶ Maxillary Universal Forceps—Cryer 150 must be precleaned open and unlocked, placed in an open and unlocked position either in a sterilizing pouch with an internal process indicator, sealed, then sterilized OR wrapped with an internal process indicator inside and secured on the outside with process indicator tape, then sterilized. Verify appropriate color change has been achieved in external process indicator immediately after removal from sterilizer then check internal process indicator before treatment. Refer to state regulations for any additional state requirements.

Mandibular Universal Forceps—Cryer 151

Function ▶ To extract mandibular centrals, laterals, cuspids, premolars, and roots

Characteristics ▶ Straight handles or one curved handle

Practice Note ▶ Mandibular Universal Forceps—Cryer 151 are used on surgical extraction tray setups.

Sterilization Notes ▶ Mandibular Universal Forceps—Cryer 151 must be precleaned open and unlocked, placed in an open and unlocked position either in a sterilizing pouch with an internal process indicator, sealed, then sterilized OR wrapped with an internal process indicator inside and secured on the outside with process indicator tape, then sterilized. Verify appropriate color change has been achieved in external process indicator immediately after removal from sterilizer then check internal process indicator before treatment. Refer to state regulations for any additional state requirements.

Mandibular Anterior Forceps

Function ▶ To extract mandibular anterior teeth

Characteristic ▶ Serrated beaks

Practice Note ▶ Mandibular Anterior Forceps are used on surgical extraction tray setups.

Sterilization Notes ▶ Mandibular Anterior Forceps must be precleaned open and unlocked, placed in an open and unlocked position either in a sterilizing pouch with an internal process indicator, sealed, then sterilized OR wrapped with an internal process indicator inside and secured on the outside with process indicator tape, then sterilized. Verify appropriate color change has been achieved in external process indicator immediately after removal from sterilizer then check internal process indicator before treatment. Refer to state regulations for any additional state requirements.

Maxillary Root Forceps

Function ▶ To extract maxillary roots

Characteristics ▶ Narrow, serrated beaks
Straight handles

Practice Note ▶ Maxillary Root Forceps are used on surgical extraction tray setups.

Sterilization Notes ▶ Maxillary Root Forceps must be precleaned open and unlocked, placed in an open and unlocked position either in a sterilizing pouch with an internal process indicator, sealed, then sterilized OR wrapped with an internal process indicator inside and secured on the outside with process indicator tape, then sterilized. Verify appropriate color change has been achieved in external process indicator immediately after removal from sterilizer then check internal process indicator before treatment. Refer to state regulations for any additional state requirements.

Mandibular Root Forceps

Function ▶ To extract mandibular roots

Characteristics ▶ Narrow, serrated beaks
Straight handles

Practice Note ▶ Mandibular Root Forceps are used on surgical extraction tray setups.

Sterilization Notes ▶ Mandibular Root Forceps must be precleaned open and unlocked, placed in an open and unlocked position either in a sterilizing pouch with an internal process indicator, sealed, then sterilized OR wrapped with an internal process indicator inside and secured on the outside with process indicator tape, then sterilized. Verify appropriate color change has been achieved in external process indicator immediately after removal from sterilizer then check internal process indicator before treatment. Refer to state regulations for any additional state requirements.

Implant System

Function ▶ To use for implant surgery

Characteristics ▶ Components—Depth drills, thread formers, hand wrench, ratchet, ratchet adapter, hex driver

Many types of implant systems available

Practice Notes ▶ Implant System is used on a surgical tray setup.

Sterile technique must be kept during procedure.

Sterilization Notes ▶ Implant System must be precleaned, either, placed in a sterilizing pouch with an internal process indicator, sealed, then sterilized OR wrapped with an internal process indicator inside and secured on the outside with process indicator tape, then sterilized. Verify appropriate color change has been achieved in external process indicator immediately after removal from sterilizer then check internal process indicator before treatment. Refer to state regulations for any additional state requirements.

Implant

Function ▶ To use for implant surgery

Characteristics ▶ Endosteal implant—An implant surgically embedded into the bone

Osseointegration—The attachment of healthy bone to a dental implant, also referred to as stably integrated

Two other types of implants—Subperiosteal and transosteal

Components:

1 Implant fixture (titanium) embedded into bone; many styles of implants available

2 Center screw

3 Crown

Practice Notes ▶ Implant is used on a surgical tray setup.

Sterile technique must be kept during procedure.

Sterilization Notes ▶ Implant must be precleaned, either, placed in a sterilizing pouch with an internal process indicator, sealed, then sterilized OR wrapped with an internal process indicator inside and secured on the outside with process indicator tape, then sterilized. Verify appropriate color change has been achieved in external process indicator immediately after removal from sterilizer then check internal process indicator before treatment. Refer to state regulations for any additional state requirements. Use a biological indicator for every sterilizer load that contains an implantable device. Whenever possible, verify results before using the implantable device, according to the Centers for Disease Control and Prevention Guidelines for Infection Control in Dental Health-Care Settings—2003, Recommendations, Category IB. Strongly recommended for implementation and supported by experimental, clinical, or epidemiologic studies and a strong theoretical rationale.

Extraction of Maxillary Right First Molar

TOP ROW (LEFT TO RIGHT)

Mouth mirror, explorer, cotton forceps, periosteal elevator, straight elevator, surgical curette, tissue forceps, hemostat, tissue scissors, mouth prop, needle holder, suture scissors, tongue and cheek retractor (Minnesota), disposable high-volume surgical evacuation tip, and maxillary right forceps no. 88R

BOTTOM ROW

Silk suture with needle in sterile package

Sterilization Notes ▶ Refer to each picture for correct procedure for instrument sterilization or disposal of instrument or material. Refer to Chapter 15 to see additional instruments used in oral surgery extractions. Also refer to other chapters for additional instruments on this tray setup that are not included in this chapter.

For mandibular first or second molar extraction, the tray setup is identical to the tray setup for the extraction of a maxillary right first molar, except that a mandibular right forceps No. 17 is used in place of a maxillary right forceps No. 88R.

Extraction of Impacted Mandibular Molar

TOP ROW (LEFT TO RIGHT)

Mouth mirror, explorer, cotton forceps (pliers), scalpel #12 with blade, periosteal elevator, straight elevator, right and left root-tip elevators, surgical curette, tissue forceps, rongeurs, bone file, surgical chisel, surgical mallet

BOTTOM ROW (LEFT TO RIGHT)

Tissue scissors, hemostat, silk suture with needle in sterile package, needle holder, suture scissors, tongue and cheek retractor (Minnesota), surgical long-shank burs in bur holder, mouth prop, disposable high-volume surgical evacuation tip, universal mandibular forceps No. 16

Sterilization Notes ▶ Refer to each picture for correct procedure for instrument sterilization or disposal of instrument or material. Refer to Chapter 15 to see additional instruments used in oral surgery extractions. Also refer to other chapters for additional instruments on this tray setup that are not included in this chapter.

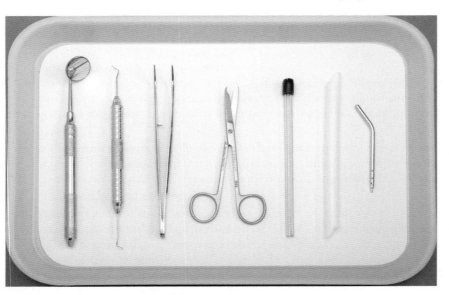

Suture Removal

LEFT TO RIGHT

Mouth mirror, pigtail explorer, cotton forceps (pliers), suture scissors, saliva ejector, high-volume evacuator (HVE) tip, air/water syringe tip

Sterilization Notes ▶ Refer to each picture for correct procedure for instrument sterilization or disposal of instrument or material. Refer to other chapters for instruments on this tray setup.

Sterilization and Protective Equipment

Protective Gown

Function ▶ To protect clothing, surgical scrubs, and skin during patient care and sterilization process to prevent contamination from blood and body substances

Characteristics ▶ Disposable (pictured) or cloth (Cloth gowns must be made of polyester and cotton in accordance with state and federal regulations.)
Cuffed long sleeves
Closure at neckline
Moisture resistant (against contamination by liquids)
Many styles available

Practice Notes ▶ All protective clothing should be removed before leaving the workplace.
Follow regulations within the state for standard precautions.

Sterilization Notes ▶ Dispose of Protective Gown in garbage at the end of the day. If lab coat becomes visibly soiled during the work day, change to a new lab coat. Cloth lab coats must be laundered each day.

Protective Mask

Functions ▶ To protect against chemicals, airborne pathogens, bacteria, and viruses during processing of instruments for sterilization

To protect against airborne pathogens, bacteria, and viruses and against scrap filling material during all phases of patient treatment

Characteristics ▶ Dome shaped or flat

Different levels of filtration

Practice Notes ▶ Protective Mask must cover nose and mouth. Protective Mask must be worn during dental procedures with a patient and during any exposure to dental material that is airborne.

Sterilization Notes ▶ Protective Mask should be disposed of in the garbage. A new mask must be used with each patient.

Protective Glasses/Loupes

Functions ▶ To protect against chemicals, airborne pathogens, bacteria, and viruses during processing of instruments for sterilization

To protect against airborne pathogens, bacteria, and viruses during patient care and against scrap-filling material during restorative and rinsing phases of patient treatment

To enhance (Loupes) depth-of-focus and field-of-view during treatment

Characteristics ▶ Extend to sides, top, and bottom of eyes for complete protection

1 Protective Glasses—Variety of styles available; some styles are larger to fit over prescription glasses.

2 Loupes—Have different levels of magnification; may have a light source attached to the glasses for regular patient treatment, as well as, availability to change the light source for sensitive material (such as composite restorations).

Practice Notes ▶ Facial shields available for eye protection (mask must be worn)

Protective glasses must be worn during dental procedures with a patient, sterilization, and during any exposure to dental material that is airborne.

Loupes allow a practitioner to maintain a more physiologic posture promoting ergonomically correct chair position during treatment.

Sterilization Notes ▶ Protective glasses/loupes are disinfected between patients according to the manufacturer's recommendation. Refer to state regulations for any additional state requirements.

▪INSTRUMENT Examination Gloves

Functions ▶ To wear during patient care
To wear as a protective barrier
To wear during treatment room disinfection

Characteristics ▶ Latex (pictured), nitrile, or vinyl — Nonsterile and sterile gloves are available.
Nonsterile gloves worn for most dental procedures; sterile gloves may be worn for surgical procedures.
Examination Gloves should be worn over cuff of protective gown.
Various sizes available

Practice Notes ▶ Examination Gloves are single use only. Wash or sanitize hands before putting on gloves and after removing gloves. Must change if leaving patient care, or use overgloves (refer to pages 590 and 591). Replace worn or torn gloves immediately (along with washing hands or using hand sanitizer [follow state guidelines]). If procedure is long, change gloves every hour. Gloves must go over cuff of lab coat.

Sterilization Notes ▶ Examination Gloves must be disposed of in the garbage.

Overgloves

Functions ▶ To wear over examination gloves when leaving the patient
To wear as a protective barrier over examination gloves so as not to cross-contaminate

Characteristics ▶ Lightweight clear gloves
Not to be worn for dental procedures
Various sizes available

Practice Notes ▶ New set of overgloves must be used for each patient. Keep overgloves in an uncontaminated area of the treatment room. Must be careful to not contaminate outside of overgloves when putting on over examination gloves.

Sterilization Notes ▶ Overgloves must be disposed of in the garbage.

Nitrile Utility Gloves

Functions ▶ To protect hands during processing of instruments for sterilization procedures
To wear for preparation and handling of chemicals
To disinfect operatory
To transport cassettes of tray setups to sterilization area from treatment area

Characteristics ▶ Chemical resistant
Puncture resistant
Ribbed for nonslip grip
Range of sizes and colors
Refer to state regulations on when utility gloves should be worn

Practice Note ▶ Nitrile Utility Gloves should be kept in sterilization area of office.

Sterilization Notes ▶ Nitrile Utility Gloves are disinfected after each use. Sterilize according to the manufacturer's recommendation and refer to local and state regulations.

Cassette

Functions ▶ To use for instruments as tray setup
To use for instrument sterilization

Characteristics ▶ Available in metal or resin
Color coded
Range of sizes

Practice Notes ▶ Instruments in the cassette may be cleaned in an ultrasonic cleaner and then wrapped and sterilized.
Color coding aids in the identification of cassettes and tray setups.

Sterilization Notes ▶ Cassette with instruments must be precleaned, either, placed in a sterilizing pouch with an internal process indicator, sealed, then sterilized OR wrapped with an internal process indicator inside and secured on the outside with process indicator tape, then sterilized. Verify appropriate color change has been achieved in external process indicator immediately after removal from sterilizer then check internal process indicator before treatment. Refer to state regulations for any additional state requirements.

Color-Coding System for Instruments

Function ▶ To color code instruments for organization and identification of tray setups

Characteristic ▶ Variety of colors—Color coding coordinates with color cassettes

Practice Note ▶ The Color-Coding System makes it easier to identify tray setups and instruments within the tray setup.

Sterilization Notes ▶ Color-Coded Instruments must be precleaned, either, placed in a sterilizing pouch with an internal process indicator, sealed, then sterilized OR wrapped with an internal process indicator inside and secured on the outside with process indicator tape, then sterilized. Verify appropriate color change has been achieved in external process indicator immediately after removal from sterilizer then check internal process indicator before treatment. Refer to state regulations for any additional state requirements.

Parts Box for Sterilization

Function ▶ To use for sterilization of small items
Examples: Burs, dental dam clamps

Characteristic ▶ Range of sizes to accommodate sterilization needs

Practice Note ▶ Parts Box helps hold and organize small items for tray setups.

Sterilization Notes ▶ Parts Box must be precleaned, either, placed in a sterilizing pouch with an internal process indicator, sealed, then sterilized OR wrapped with an internal process indicator inside and secured on the outside with process indicator tape, then sterilized. Verify appropriate color change has been achieved in external process indicator immediately after removal from sterilizer then check internal process indicator before treatment. Refer to state regulations for any additional state requirements.

▪INSTRUMENT Cassette Wrap

Functions ▶ To use to wrap cassette during sterilization
To store cassette in wrapping after sterilization
To use for tray cover during dental procedure

Characteristic ▶ Range of sizes—To accommodate cassettes

Practice Note ▶ Cassettes should be kept in sterile wrap until the patient is seated. Refer to local and state regulations.

Sterilization Notes ▶ All instruments or cassettes must be precleaned, either, placed in a sterilizing pouch with an internal process indicator, sealed, then sterilized OR wrapped with an internal process indicator inside and secured on the outside with process indicator tape, then sterilized. Verify appropriate color change has been achieved in external process indicator immediately after removal from sterilizer then write date and sterilizer used on wrap. Check internal process indicator before treatment. Refer to state regulations for any additional state requirements.

·INSTRUMENT Sterilization Pouches

Function ▶ To be used for sterilization of instruments and cassettes

Characteristic ▶ Pouches have range of sizes to accommodate all sizes of instruments and cassettes.

Available with Self Seal Pouches

Available with indicator strip on pouch

1 Indicator strip changed color after sterilization

2 Indicator strip color before sterilization

3 Cassette with indicator tape on outside of pouch

Practice Note ▶ Instruments should be kept in the pouches until the patient is seated. Refer to state regulations.

Sterilization Notes ▶ All instruments must be precleaned placed in a sterilization pouch with an internal process indicator, sealed, then sterilized. Verify appropriate color change has been achieved in external process indicator immediately after removal from sterilizer then write date and sterilizer used on pouch. Check internal process indicator before treatment. Refer to state regulations for any additional state requirements.

■INSTRUMENT   Indicator Tape and Dispensing Unit

Functions ▶ To secure wrap on outside of cassette

To use outside cassettes or sterilization pouches to indicate exposure of instruments to a certain temperature—Color will change on the tape.

Characteristics ▶ Available in preprinted tray setup procedures-refer to page 602 and 603.

Available with color coding

Available blank for labeling tape with procedure and/or instrument content

Practice Note ▶ Instruments should be kept in the pouches until the patient is seated. Refer to state regulations.

Sterilization Notes ▶ When Indicator Tape is placed outside a cassette, the strips change color with exposure to temperature of the sterilization process; they do not determine the actual sterilization. Refer to sterilization monitoring. If the indicator tape does not change color the pouch or wrap must be resterilized.

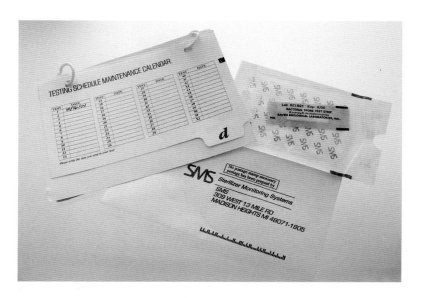

■INSTRUMENT Biological Monitors for Sterilizers

Function ▶ To confirm efficacy of sterilization, documentation of results is recorded in office sterilization log

Characteristic ▶ Many systems available

Practice Note ▶ Biological Monitor Testing device is placed in the sterilizer for one cycle of instruments. It is then mailed to the manufacturer, which mails back the findings. The results are logged in the office sterilization records.

Sterilization Notes ▶ The Centers for Disease Control and Prevention, the American Dental Association, and the Office Safety and Asepsis Procedures Research Foundation recommend at least weekly testing of each sterilizer in the office. Local and state requirements may be different.

◾INSTRUMENT Sterilization Spore Check—In Office

Function ▸ To monitor and confirm the effectiveness of steam sterilizers

Characteristics ▸
1. Record book
2. Self-contained biological indicator
3. Dry block incubator

Practice Note ▸ A vial with the solution is marked and placed in a sterilization pouch, and the sterilization cycle is processed. After the cycle is complete, follow the directions; then place vial in incubator. Results will occur in 24 hours. Record results.

Sterilization Notes ▸ Steam sterilizers should be checked for effectiveness every week. Every load of implants should be monitored for effectiveness when possible with each implant before each implant procedure.

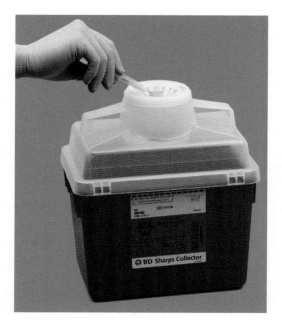

Sharps Container

Function ▶ To serve as storage receptacle for used needles, old burs, scalpel blades, orthodontic wires, endodontic files, and all other disposable sharp items used during dental procedures

Characteristics ▶ Must be puncture resistant
Must be labeled "Biohazard"
Must have a reclosable top

Practice Note ▶ Sharps containers must be disposed of according to local, state, and federal regulations and by an Environmental Protection Agency regulatory disposal company. Required paperwork must be kept according to state and federal regulations.

Sterilization Notes ▶ Refer to state and local regulations on the type of glove (utility and patient glove) to handle sharps that are disposed in the Sharps Container.

Ultrasonic Cleaning Unit

Function ▶ To remove debris and bioburden from instruments

Characteristic ▶ Reduces risk of exposure to pathogens during the cleaning stage of the sterilization process

Practice Notes ▶ Tank is filled with antimicrobial or general all-purpose solution specially designed for the ultrasonic unit. Fill and drain solution daily.

Debris is removed by mechanical means; sound waves create tiny bubbles that cause inward collapse (implosion) and removal of material. Lid must be closed during operation of unit. Available in some units are racks for cassettes.

Sterilization Notes ▶ After cleaning the instruments in the ultrasonic cleaning unit, instruments must be rinsed and either be placed in a sterilizing pouch with an internal process indicator, sealed, then sterilized OR wrapped with an internal process indicator inside and secured on the outside with process indicator tape, then sterilized. Verify appropriate color change has been achieved in external process indicator immediately after removal from sterilizer then check internal process indicator before treatment. Refer to state regulations for any additional state requirements. For precleaning instruments *Guidelines for Infection Control in Dental Health-Care Settings—2003* states "that the use of automated cleaning equipment such as ultrasonic cleaner or washer-disinfector is safer than hand scrubbing instruments prior to continuing the sterilization process even though hand washing is acceptable."

▪INSTRUMENT Sterilizer—Autoclave (Saturated Steam)

Function ▶ To kill all microbes, viruses, bacteria, and fungi, thereby sterilizing instruments

Characteristics ▶ Uses steam under pressure—15 pounds per square inch (psi) at 250°F for 20 minutes
Shelves and racks are available for cassettes
Various styles and manufacturers
Range of sizes

Practice Notes ▶ Refer to federal, state, and manufacturer's sterilization techniques as well as manufacturer's maintenance requirements.

Sterilization Notes ▶ The Centers for Disease Control and Prevention, the American Dental Association, and the Office Safety and Asepsis Procedures Research Foundation recommend at least weekly testing of Sterilizers. Local and state requirements may be different. Refer to pages 606 and 607 for Biological Monitors for Sterilization.

Statim G4 Cassette Autoclave

Functions ▶ To kill all microbes, viruses, bacteria, and fungi
To sterilize instruments and handpieces

Characteristics ▶ Statim 2000 G4 cycle times: 6 minutes unwrapped, 14 minutes wrapped
Statim 5000 G4 cycle times: 9 minutes unwrapped, 17.5 minutes wrapped
Uses fresh steam-distilled water with every cycle
Uses Dri-Tec drying system for fast dry loads
Readout Screen available for each cycle

Practice Note ▶ Refer to federal, state, and manufacturer's sterilization techniques as well as manufacturer's maintenance requirements.

Sterilization Notes ▶ The Centers for Disease Control and Prevention, the American Dental Association, and the Office Safety and Asepsis Procedures Research Foundation recommend at least weekly testing of sterilizers. Local and state requirements may be different. Refer to pages 606 and 607 for Biological Monitors for Sterilization.

▪INSTRUMENT Sterilizer—Dry Heat (Static Air)

Function ▶ To kill all microbes, viruses, bacteria, and fungi, thereby sterilizing instruments

Characteristics ▶ Oven-type sterilizer
320°F for 60 to 120 minutes
Shelves available for cassettes
Various styles and manufacturers
Range of sizes

Practice Notes ▶ Packaging and wrapped material must be able to withstand high temperatures.
Door cannot be opened during sterilization cycle.
Items cannot be layered or stacked but should be placed on their edges.

Sterilization Notes ▶ The Centers for Disease Control and Prevention, the American Dental Association, and the Office Safety and Asepsis Procedures Research Foundation recommend at least weekly testing of Sterilizers. Local and state requirements may be different. Refer to pages 606 and 607 for Biological Monitors for Sterilization.

■INSTRUMENT Sterilizer—Dry Heat (Rapid Heat Transfer)

Function ▸ To kill all microbes, viruses, bacteria, and fungi, thereby sterilizing instruments

Characteristics ▸ Forced air–type sterilizer
375°F for 12 minutes (wrapped)
375°F for 6 minutes (unwrapped)
Instruments placed in preheated chamber
Various styles and manufacturers
Range of sizes

Practice Notes ▸ Packaging and wrapped material must be able to withstand high temperatures.
Door cannot be opened during sterilization cycle.

Sterilization Notes ▸ The Centers for Disease Control and Prevention, the American Dental Association, and the Office Safety and Asepsis Procedures Research Foundation recommend at least weekly testing of Sterilizers. Local and state requirements may be different. Refer to pages 606 and 607 for Biological Monitors for Sterilization.

Dental Materials Equipment

Flexible Rubber Bowl

Functions ▶ To mix material, usually a powder and a liquid

To mix impression material and irreversible hydrocolloid for study models, opposing models, bleaching trays, night guards, mouth guards, orthodontic appliances, or custom trays for removable appliances

To mix laboratory plaster, stone, and die stone for models

Characteristic ▶ Bowl is flexible to manipulate material.

Practice Note ▶ Flexible Rubber Bowl is used with the alginate spatula.

Sterilization Notes ▶ Preclean and disinfect Flexible Rubber Bowl before and after each use according to the manufacturer's recommendation.

Flexible Alginate (Irreversible Hydrocolloid) Spatula

Functions ▶ To mix powder and a liquid in a flexible bowl
To mix impression material such as irreversible hydrocolloid (alginate)
To mix laboratory plaster, stone, and die stone for models

Characteristic ▶ Spatula is flexible to manipulate material.

Practice Note ▶ Flexible Alginate Spatula is used with the flexible rubber bowl.

Sterilization Notes ▶ Preclean and disinfect Flexible Alginate Spatula before and after each use according to manufacturer's recommendation.

INSTRUMENT ## Disposable Plastic Perforated Full Arch Impression Trays

Function ▶ To use for taking impressions with many types of impression material
Example: Irreversible hydrocolloid (alginate), crown, and bridge impression material

Characteristics ▶
1 Maxillary perforated tray
2 Mandibular perforated tray

Perforated trays allow material to push through the tray, creating a mechanical lock that keeps the material in place.
Range of sizes

Practice Notes ▶ Disposable Plastic Perforated trays are used for many types of dental procedures involving taking impressions.
Impressions must be rinsed then disinfected before pouring up impressions.

Sterilization Notes ▶ Disposable Plastic Perforated Full Arch Impression Trays should be disposed of in the garbage. Single use only.

Metal Perforated Full Arch Impression Trays

Function ▶ To use for taking impressions with many types of impression material.
Example: Irreversible hydrocolloid (alginate), crown, and bridge impression material

Characteristics ▶ **1** Maxillary Metal Perforated Tray
2 Mandibular Metal Perforated Tray

Perforated trays allow material to push through the tray, creating a mechanical lock that keeps the material in place.
Range of sizes

Practice Notes ▶ Metal Perforated Full Arch Impression Trays are used for many types of dental procedures involving taking impressions.
Impression trays must be rinsed then disinfected before pouring up impressions.

Sterilization Notes ▶ Metal Perforated Full Arch Impression Trays must be precleaned, either, placed in a sterilizing pouch with an internal process indicator, sealed, then sterilized OR wrapped with an internal process indicator inside and secured on the outside with process indicator tape, then sterilized. Verify appropriate color change has been achieved in external process indicator immediately after removal from sterilizer then check internal process indicator before treatment. Refer to state regulations for any additional state requirements.

▪INSTRUMENT Disposable Plastic Perforated Quadrant and Anterior Impression Trays

Functions ▶ To use for taking impressions with many types of impression material
To use for taking a quadrant or anterior portion of the mouth

Characteristics ▶
1 Section tray for anterior maxillary or mandibular perforated tray
2 Maxillary left or mandibular right perforated tray
3 Maxillary right or mandibular left perforated tray

Perforated trays allow material to push through the tray, creating a mechanical lock that keeps the material in place.
Range of sizes
Metal quadrant and anterior trays also available. Refer to sterilization notes below.

Practice Notes ▶ Disposable Plastic Perforated Quadrant and Anterior Impression Trays are used for many types of dental procedures involving taking impressions.
Impressions must be rinsed then disinfected before pouring up impressions.

Sterilization Notes ▶ Disposable Plastic Perforated Quadrant And Anterior Impression Trays should be disposed of in the garbage. Single use only.

Alginator

Function ▶ To mix alginate, irreversible hydrocolloid automatically

Characteristics ▶ Flexible bowl attaches to alginator
Low and high buttons allow bowl to rotate, mixing the alginate and water together.
Spatula pressing the material against the bowl along with the rotation of the bowl results in the material being a smooth consistency.

Practice Notes ▶ Alginator is used for many dental procedures involving taking an alginate impression.
Impressions must be cleaned and disinfected before pouring up impressions.

Sterilization Notes ▶ Alginator case must be precleaned, sprayed with a disinfectant to wipe clean the surface, then, sprayed a second time to disinfect according the manufacturers guidelines with an approved TB/hospital wipe or spray. The Flexible Alginate Bowl must be precleaned thoroughly after removing alginate from the bowl, then, sprayed a second time to disinfect with an approved TB/hospital wipe or spray. Switch on the unit when wiping the bowl to assure thorough coverage. Refer to state regulations for any additional state requirements.

Triple Tray (Disposable)

Functions ▶ To use for taking final impressions for crown and bridge restorations, opposing teeth, and bite registration with one impression
To use in the mouth, taking maxillary and mandibular simultaneously
To use with many types of impression material

Characteristics ▶ Trays have a ledge on the side to hold sufficient amount of material for the impression.
Trays have mesh-type material in the middle of the tray to hold material in place.
Trays available:
- Quadrant used for maxillary right/left or mandibular right/left
- Maxillary left or mandibular right perforated tray
- Anterior maxillary or mandibular perforated tray

Practice Note ▶ Triple Trays are used for many types of dental procedures.
Impressions must be rinsed then disinfected before pouring up impressions.

Sterilization Notes ▶ Triple Trays should be disposed of in the garbage. Single use only.

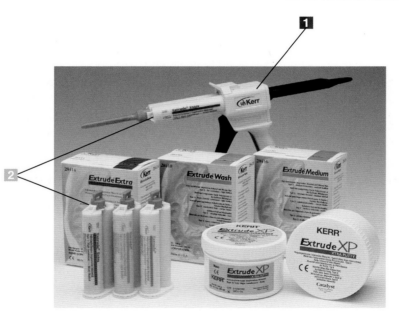

Mixing Gun for Dental Impression Material

Functions ▶ To mix polyvinylsiloxane, polysulfide, and polyether material for final impression
To mix base and catalyst for impression tray
To mix wash material for the syringe
To mix material for bite registration and temporary crowns

Characteristics ▶ **1** Mixing gun
2 Material used in gun

Manufacturers have different-style guns to accommodate their material.
A different technique for the tray material is to mix a putty material that is a base and a catalyst.

Practice Notes ▶ A tube with the base and catalyst is inserted into the mixing gun with a mixing rod attached.
Pressure is placed on the trigger of the gun, and the material extrudes from the tubes into the mixing rod and onto the impression tray or into the tube of the syringe.
Tray material and wash (syringe) material are different.

Sterilization Notes ▶ Use overgloves to handle Mixing Gun or preclean and disinfect after each use according to the manufacturer's recommendation. Mixing rod tips should be disposed of in the garbage. Single use only.

Automixer

Functions ▶ To automatically mix impression material
To mix base and catalyst for polyvinylsiloxane and polyether
material
To place material after dispensing from automixer into
impression trays for final impressions

Characteristics ▶ Different styles of automixers available
Must attach mixing tips

Practice Notes ▶ A wash material (delivered from a syringe) is placed on the
prepared tooth by the operator before the tray with the
impression material is placed in the patient's mouth.
Polyvinylsiloxane can also be mixed manually.

Sterilization Notes ▶ Use overgloves to handle Automixer or preclean and disinfect after each use according to the
manufacturer's recommendation.

Bite Registration Tray

Functions ▶ To use for taking bite registration for crown and bridge procedures
To use in the mouth, taking maxillary and mandibular simultaneously
To use with many types of bite registration material

Characteristics ▶ Trays have mesh-type material in the middle of the tray to hold material in place.
Range of sizes
Trays can be used in right or left quadrant.
Anterior section bite registration tray is also available.

Practice Notes ▶ Bite Registration Trays is used with crown and bridge tray setup.
Mixing guns may be used to mix material.
Bite registration tray should be rinsed then disinfected before sending to laboratory.

Sterilization Notes ▶ Bite Registration Trays should be disposed of in the garbage.
Single use only.

Reversible Hydrocolloid Unit

Function ▶ To boil reversible hydrocolloid, store, and temper material for final impressions

Characteristics ▶ Hydrocolloid unit has three baths:

1 Liquefying the semisolid material at 212°F (100°C)
2 Storage bath that cools the material and keeps it ready for impressions at 150°F (65.5°C)
3 Tempering bath holds the filled impression tray for 5 minutes before it is placed in the patient's mouth at 110°F (44°C).

Tubes of the material are for the impression tray.
Small cylinders are for the wash material and are used in syringes for operator to place around tooth before impression is taken.

Practice Note ▶ Reversible hydrocolloid water-cooled impression trays need to be used for this type of impression material.

Sterilization Notes ▶ Preclean and disinfect Reversible Hydrocolloid Unit, if contaminated, before and after each use according to the manufacturer's recommendation.

Reversible Hydrocolloid Water-Cooled Impression Trays and Hose

Function ▸ To take impression with reversible hydrocolloid

Characteristics ▸
1 Mandibular water-cooled tray
2 Maxillary water-cooled tray
3 Attaches to tray
4 Attaches to water source on dental unit
5 Attaches to vacuum system of dental unit

A hose attaches to the tray on one end; the other end attaches to a water source and a vacuum for the water. The water runs inside the tray, which cools and sets the material once in the patient's mouth.

Practice Note ▸ Important to connect all parts of the hose before turning on the water source
Impression must be rinsed then disinfected before sending to lab

Sterilization Notes ▸ Irreversible Hydrocolloid Water-cooled Impression Trays must be precleaned, either, placed in a sterilizing pouch with an internal process indicator, sealed, then sterilized OR wrapped with an internal process indicator inside and secured on the outside with process indicator tape, then sterilized. Verify appropriate color change has been achieved in external process indicator immediately after removal from sterilizer then check internal process indicator before treatment. Refer to state regulations for any additional state requirements. Hose must be precleaned and disinfected according to the manufacturer's recommendation.

Laboratory Spatula

Functions ▶ To mix powder and a liquid in a flexible bowl
To mix and shape laboratory plaster, stone, and die
stone for models

Characteristics ▶ Spatula straight to help manipulate material
Range of sizes

Practice Note ▶ Laboratory Spatula is used with vibrator.

Sterilization Notes ▶ Preclean and disinfect Laboratory Spatula, if
contaminated, after each use according to the
manufacturer's recommendation. Refer to state
regulations for any additional state requirements.

Vibrator for Laboratory

Function ▶ To vibrate material in mixing bowl to remove air bubbles from mixing plaster, stone, or die stone

Characteristics ▶ Use vibrator after mixing the plaster or stone. Use vibrator while adding plaster or stone to impression to eliminate air bubbles in impression.

Practice Note ▶ Place plastic cover on vibrator work surface to keep vibrator free from material.

Sterilization Notes ▶ Preclean and disinfect vibrator, if contaminated, according to the manufacturer's recommendation.

Vacuum Mixing Unit

Functions ▶ To vacuum mix all types of gypsums, plasters, and investment materials
To program digitally type of material being mixed
To remove excessive air from material while mixing

Characteristics ▶ Vacuum mixing unit uses blades to mix material and vacuums air bubbles
Bowl with blades attaches to unit and mixes material automatically
Vacuum system within the unit removes excess air for smoother material consistency

Practice Note ▶ Vacuum Mixer used in dental office labs and dental laboratories for better consistency of
material for models and investment material for cast crowns.

Sterilization Notes ▶ Preclean and disinfect Vacuum Mixing Unit and Mixing Bowls, if contaminated, according
to manufacturer's recommendation.

Laboratory Knife

Functions ▶ To use for separating impressions from model(s)
To use for hand-trimming models
To use on any type of appliance for hand trimming

Characteristics ▶ Range of sizes
Usually has green wooden handle—Referred to as Green Handle Lab Knife

Practice Note ▶ Laboratory Knife is used in dental office setting and dental laboratories.

Sterilization Notes ▶ Preclean and disinfect Laboratory Knife, if contaminated, according to manufacturer's recommendation. Refer to state regulations for any additional state requirements.

Model Trimmer

Function ▶ To trim plaster, stone, or die stone models

Characteristics ▶ Trimmer has an abrasive grinding wheel to grind excess plaster, stone, and die stone from the models.
Water runs next to the grinding wheel to reduce heat, reduce the dust created by grinding, and keep the wheel clean.

Practice Notes ▶ Diagnostic models, orthodontic models, and crown and bridge models are all trimmed differently.
Glasses and mask should be worn while trimming models.
Unit should have splash guards.

Sterilization Notes ▶ Preclean and disinfect Model Trimmer, if contaminated, according to the manufacturer's recommendation.

Flexible Mixing Spatula

Function ▶ To mix dental materials

Characteristics ▶ Flexible metal to allow proper manipulation
Range of sizes

Practice Note ▶ Flexible Mixing Spatula is used on most restorative, endodontic, orthodontic, and periodontic tray setups.

Sterilization Notes ▶ Flexible Mixing Spatula must be precleaned, either, placed in a sterilizing pouch with an internal process indicator, sealed, then sterilized OR wrapped with an internal process indicator inside and secured on the outside with process indicator tape, then sterilized. Verify appropriate color change has been achieved in external process indicator immediately after removal from sterilizer then check internal process indicator before treatment. Refer to state regulations for any additional state requirements.

Paper Mixing Pads

Function ▶ To mix all types of dental materials

Characteristics ▶ Each paper on the pad is coated so material will not seep through the paper.
Many types and sizes available

Practice Note ▶ Many materials have special paper pads that must be used when mixing certain materials.

Sterilization Notes ▶ Remove one paper to mix each material and not contaminate the pad. Entire pad should not be used to mix unless overgloves are used.

Dental Imaging and Diagnostic Equipment

OPPOSITE SIDE
TOWARD TUBE
Kodak
INSIGHT
Dental Film

Intraoral Dental Film

Function ▶ To capture the image of teeth in the radiographic process

Characteristics ▶
1. Outside covering of film—Soft plastic or paper (both waterproof)
2. Sheet of lead foil to stop the radiation from extending beyond the film
3. Black paper to protect the film from light penetration
4. Film—Single or double film

Film speed indicated on each packet—Set by American National Standards Institute (ANSI)
Film speed A through F—D, E, F used intraorally
Faster speed of the film reduces the amount of radiation exposure; F speed is faster than D speed.
Film speed determines amount of radiation needed to produce a quality radiograph—Settings are on x-ray unit.

Practice Note ▶ Intraoral Dental X-ray Film is used in all phases of dentistry.

Sterilization Notes ▶ Follow standard precautions and cross-contamination protocol when exposing and processing film for developing. Outer packet and black paper may be disposed of in the garbage. Correct disposal of lead foil must be checked within your state. In some states, lead foil is considered a hazardous waste and must be collected and disposed of properly. For proper recycling protocol, refer to Department of Environmental Health regulations in the state where you practice.

Intraoral Dental Film—Various Sizes

Functions ▶ To project an image of the patient's teeth through x-ray onto the film
To use for intraoral and extraoral projections

Characteristics ▶ Commonly taken radiographs—Front and back view
Size #0—Taken on children under 3 (not pictured)

1 Size #1—Used for Anterior periapical image (narrow view)

2 Size #2—Used for Periapical and bite-wing image

Size #3—Used for extended bitewing projections (not pictured)

3 Size #4—Used for occlusal projections; taken to view maxillary and mandibular teeth; commonly taken on children

Practice Notes ▶ Smooth side of the film (the raised-dot side—convex) faces the x-ray tube or position-indicating device (PID). Raised dot should be toward the occlusal or incisal.

Sterilization Notes ▶ Follow standard precautions and cross-contamination protocol when exposing and processing film for developing. Outer packet and black paper may be disposed of in the garbage. Correct disposal of lead foil must be checked within your state. In some states, lead foil is considered a hazardous waste and must be collected and disposed of properly. For proper recycling protocol, refer to Department of Environmental Health regulations in the state where you practice. Refer to state regulations for any additional state requirements.

Package of Dental Film

Function ▶ To package intraoral dental film

Characteristics ▶ Box labeled:
- Type of film
- Film speed
- Number of films in individual film packet
- Number of film packets in the box
- Expiration date of film

Film packets—Single or double film

Practice Notes ▶ Each film has an identification dot (raised bump). Concave on one side and convex on the other. Convex/bump faces toward the teeth when placing the x-ray.

Film storage is important to the integrity of the film. Refer to package instructions for storage recommendations.

Sterilization Notes ▶ Follow standard precautions and cross-contamination protocol when processing film for developing. Outer packet and black paper may be disposed of in the garbage. Correct disposal of lead foil must be checked within your state. In some states, lead foil is considered a hazardous waste and must be collected and disposed of properly. For proper recycling protocol, refer to Department of Environmental Health regulations in the state where you practice.

▪INSTRUMENT Bite-Wing Tabs

Function ▸ To take a bite-wing radiograph projection

Characteristics ▸ **1** Stick-on tab
2 Slip-on tab

Tab or wing is placed on the occlusal, and patient bites on the tab to secure the film.

Practice Notes ▸ Slip-on tabs are available in different sizes to accommodate different-sized film.
Size #2 film is used for adult bite-wing radiograph.
Bite-wing radiographs are mainly used for diagnosing caries on proximal surfaces (mesial and distal) of the posterior teeth.
Four bite-wings are usually taken on adult dentition—One premolar and one molar projection on each side of the mouth.

Sterilization Notes ▸ Follow standard precautions and cross-contamination protocol when exposing and processing film. Outer packet, black paper, and Bite-Wing Tabs may be disposed of in the garbage. Correct disposal of lead foil must be checked within your state. In some states, lead foil is considered a hazardous waste and must be collected and disposed of properly. For proper recycling protocol, refer to Department of Environmental Health regulations in the state where you practice.

Film Holder—Periapical (EeZee-Grip)

Function ▶ To position and hold the film in patient's mouth for periapical images

Characteristics ▶ Double ended:
- One end holds film for posterior teeth projection, as shown.
- Opposite end holds film for anterior teeth projection.

Practice Notes ▶ Size #2 film used for posterior periapical image
Size #1 or #2 used for anterior periapical image
Periapical images used for viewing the coronal part of the tooth, root, apex, and surrounding bone and tissue
EeZee-Grip formerly called Snap-a-ray

Sterilization Notes ▶ EeZee-Grip Film Holder must be precleaned open and unlocked, placed in an open and unlocked position either in a sterilizing pouch with an internal process indicator, sealed, then sterilized OR wrapped with an internal process indicator inside and secured on the outside with process indicator tape, then sterilized. Verify appropriate color change has been achieved in external process indicator immediately after removal from sterilizer then check internal process indicator before treatment. Refer to state regulations for any additional state requirements.

1
2
3

Film Holders—Periapical

Functions ▶ To position and hold a film in patient's mouth for periapical image

To allow patient to bite on holder to keep film in place while positioning the position-indicating device (PID) and exposing the film

Characteristics ▶

1 Holds film for anterior teeth projection—Plastic that can be sterilized

2 Holds film for posterior teeth projection—Plastic that can be sterilized

3 Holds film for anterior and posterior projection—Disposable Styrofoam (one time use)

Slot holds film in place

Practice Note ▶ Periapical images are used for viewing the coronal part of the tooth, root, apex, and surrounding bone and tissue.

Sterilization Notes ▶ Plastic Film Holders must be precleaned, either, placed in a sterilizing pouch with an internal process indicator, sealed, then sterilized OR wrapped with an internal process indicator inside and secured on the outside with process indicator tape, then sterilized. Verify appropriate color change has been achieved in external process indicator immediately after removal from sterilizer then check internal process indicator before treatment. Refer to state regulations for any additional state requirements. Disposable Styrofoam holder may be disposed of in garbage.

Film Holders—XCP

Functions ▶ To position and hold a film in patient's mouth for periapical and bite-wing images using parallel technique

To allow patient to bite on holder to keep film in place while positioning the position-indicating device (PID) and exposing the film

Characteristics ▶
1. Blue—Anterior teeth projection
2. Red—Bite-wing projection
3. Yellow—Posterior teeth projection
4. Green—Projections for endodontic procedures

Slot holds film in place.

Practice Notes ▶ XCP uses the parallel technique for exposing radiation to the film.
PID is parallel with the ring on the XCP.

Sterilization Notes ▶ Film Holders must be precleaned, either, placed in a sterilizing pouch with an internal process indicator, sealed, then sterilized OR wrapped with an internal process indicator inside and secured on the outside with process indicator tape, then sterilized. Verify appropriate color change has been achieved in external process indicator immediately after removal from sterilizer then check internal process indicator before treatment. Refer to state regulations for any additional state requirements.

Lead Aprons

Function ▶ To place on patient for protection against scattered x-rays during exposure of x-ray film

Characteristics ▶ **1** Lead apron
2 Lead apron with collar to protect thyroid area
3 Lead apron poncho for front and back protection

Practice Notes ▶ Lead Apron must be used when exposing patient to dental x-rays.

Lead aprons should not be folded.

Sterilization Notes ▶ Preclean and disinfect Lead Apron according to the manufacturer's recommendation.

Radiation Monitoring Device

Functions ▶ To place on operator's protective clothing while employee is working in a dental office or radiography lab

To use as a Direct Ion Storage, DIS, dosimeter constructed with non-volatile analog memory cells surround by gas-filled ion chambers

To measure the ionizing radiation exposure dose incident on the dosimeter by calculating the amount of proportional change in the voltage across the memory cells

Characteristics ▶ Each badge includes employee's name, wear and account number, and the radiation monitoring device (dosimeter).

Radiography monitoring device should be worn for traditional and digital projections.

Practice Note ▶ At the end of a reporting period, or anytime the user wants to check the dose reading on-demand, the dosimeter radiation exposure report can be read instantly and automatically via a mobile device app, localized reader, or computer. The user can also set up high-dose notification alerts or configure badge reassignments online.

Sterilization Notes ▶ If contaminated, disinfect Radiation Monitoring Device according to the manufacturer's recommendation. Refer to state regulations for any additional state requirements.

Dental X-Ray Unit

Function ▶ To expose film with radiation that is generated in the x-ray unit

Characteristics ▶
- **1** Position-indicating device (PID)
- **2** Tube head
- **3** X-ray unit

Round or rectangular PIDs available

Practice Note ▶ Control panel for the x-ray unit and button to expose the film are outside patient's treatment room. On some machines, you may adjust the exposure time the x-ray is exposed. Other machines adjust the exposure time, kilovoltage peak (kVp), and milliamperage (mA).

Sterilization Notes ▶ Follow standard precautions and cross-contamination protocol when exposing and processing film. Barriers should be used on x-ray tube head, PID, and panel where x-ray button is pushed. Follow manufacturer's recommendation for precleaning and disinfection of the Dental X-Ray Unit. Refer to state regulations for any additional state requirements.

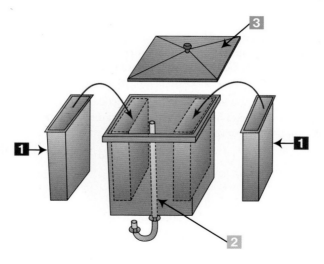

Manual Developing Unit

Functions ▶ To manually develop exposed dental radiographic films taken on patients
To develop, rinse, fix, and wash dental radiographic films
To develop dental radiographic films in a darkroom with only a safelight

Characteristics ▶ **1** Tank insert for the developing and fixing solution

Developer in left tank; fixer in right tank

2 Water bath and rinsing tank with constant running water in tank

3 Cover for unit

Practice Note ▶ Developing time depends on the temperature of the running water. The water will determine the temperature of the developer and fixer solutions. A table with the temperature denotes the time to develop and fix. Fixer time is double the developing time. The wash time is 20 minutes after the film has been fixed.

Sterilization Notes ▶ Follow standard precautions and cross-contamination protocol when processing film. For proper recycling protocol for solutions, refer to Department of Environmental Health regulations in the state where you practice. Follow local and state regulations in disposal of developer and fixer solution.

Film Rack

Functions ▶ To place undeveloped film on the rack in the darkroom with only the safelight before putting rack in the developer

To place film on rack without touching each other

Characteristic ▶ **1** Panoramic rack

2 Individual single film racks

Various sizes of racks available

Practice Note ▶ Keep films on rack through the entire process: develop, rinse, fix, wash, and dry.

Sterilization Notes ▶ Follow standard precautions and cross-contamination protocol when processing film. Outer packet and black paper may be disposed of in the garbage. Correct disposal of lead foil must be checked within your state. In some states, lead foil is considered a hazardous waste and must be collected and disposed of properly. For proper recycling protocol, refer to Department of Environmental Health regulations in the state where you practice. Disinfect racks according to manufacturer's recommendation. Refer to state regulations for any additional state requirements.

Safelight

Function ▶ To provide enough illumination in the darkroom to process films safely without exposing or damaging the film

Characteristics ▶
1 Safelight
2 Safelight filter
3 Minimum distance (at least 4 feet) from safelight to undeveloped x-ray
4 Working area
5 Undeveloped and unwrapped film

Practice Note ▶ Unwrapped film left too close to the safelight or exposed for more than 2 to 3 minutes will appear fogged.

Sterilization Notes ▶ Follow standard precautions and cross-contamination protocol when processing film. Preclean and disinfect area if contaminated.

Automatic Film Processor

Functions ▸ To automatically develop x-ray film in darkroom
To develop x-ray film

Characteristics ▸ **1** Automatic processor

2 Front loader—Hands go into a dark area to unwrap film. View area from top. Darkroom not needed.

Various types of processors available

Practice Note ▸ Dentist is able to diagnose x-ray film once film is dry, which is a great advantage of an automatic processor.

Sterilization Notes ▸ Follow standard precautions and cross-contamination protocol when processing film. Outer packet and black paper may be disposed of in the garbage. Correct disposal of lead foil must be checked within your state. In some states, lead foil is considered a hazardous waste and must be collected and disposed of properly. For proper recycling protocol, refer to Department of Environmental Health regulations in the state where you practice. Follow local and state regulations in disposal of developer and fixer solution. Refer to state regulations for any additional state requirements.

Parts of Automatic Film Processor

Functions ▶ To automatically develop x-ray film
To place film in processor to develop, fix, wash, dry; film then ready to mount

Characteristics ▶
1 Slot to feed film
2 Roller transporter in developer tank
3 Roller transporter in fixer tank
4 Roller transporter in water tank
5 Roller transporter in drying compartment
6 Film releases from rollers onto recovery slot
7 Pump to replenish developer and fixer
8 Replenishing solution for developer and fixer

Practice Note ▶ Developer and fixer solutions for the automatic processor are different from those for manual processing.

Sterilization Notes ▶ Follow standard precautions and cross-contamination protocol when processing film. Outer packet and black paper may be disposed of in the garbage. Correct disposal of lead foil must be checked within your state. In some states, lead foil is considered a hazardous waste and must be collected and disposed of properly. For proper recycling protocol for solutions, refer to Department of Environmental Health regulations in the state where you practice. Follow local and state regulations in disposal of developer and fixer solution. Refer to state regulations for any additional state requirements.

View Luminator

Function ▶	To view traditional radiographs for diagnosis
Characteristics ▶	Various sizes and styles of view luminators Also referred to as view box
Practice Note ▶	View boxes are located in each patient treatment room.
Sterilization Notes ▶	If contaminated, preclean and disinfect View Luminator according to the manufacturer's recommendation.

▪INSTRUMENT Film Duplicator

Function ▸ To duplicate dental radiographic film

Characteristics ▸ Produces white light to expose film
Various sizes and styles available

Practice Notes ▸ All phases of dentistry use film duplicators. Some dental offices use double-pack dental radiographic film instead of duplicating the film.
Electronic devices are available for duplicating dental radiographs.
Duplicated films are sent to insurance companies or referring specialists. If using double-packet dental radiographic film or digital radiography, duplication is not necessary.

Sterilization Notes ▸ If contaminated, preclean and disinfect Film Duplicator according to the manufacturer's recommendation.

■INSTRUMENT Intraoral Sensors for Digital Images

Functions ▶ To take digital intraoral images without film or without processing the film
To project the image of the teeth by digitally projecting radiation onto an electronic sensor and to computerized imaging system before going to computer storage

Characteristics ▶ Different styles and systems of sensors and digital radiography available
Different size sensors available: sizes 1, 2, and 3

1 Some sensors have wire connecting to the computer.

2 Some sensors do not have wire but are put into a specially designed computer after exposure. Picture shows barrier placed on sensor.

Practice Notes ▶ Paperless dental offices store digital x-rays on the computer, along with patient records.
Digital image may be printed out on special paper if a copy is required.
Barriers for sensors (refer to image 2 on page 698)

Sterilization Notes ▶ Follow standard precautions and cross-contamination protocol when exposing digital film. Barriers must be placed on the sensors. Barriers must be used and the manufacturer's recommendation for disinfection followed. Refer to state regulations for any additional state requirements.

Holder for Digital Sensor (EeZee-Grip)

Function ▶ To position and hold a digital x-ray sensor in patient's mouth for periapical images

Characteristics ▶ Double ended:

1 Holds film for anterior teeth projection — barrier placed on sensor

2 Holds film for posterior teeth projection — barrier placed on sensor

Designed for snug fit to prevent slipping

Practice Notes ▶ Holder allows room for the wire attached to the sensor
May be used with wireless digital sensor

Sterilization Notes ▶ Follow standard precautions and cross-contamination protocol when taking digital images. Holder must be precleaned open and unlocked, placed in an open and unlocked position either in a sterilizing pouch with an internal process indicator, sealed, then sterilized OR wrapped with an internal process indicator inside and secured on the outside with process indicator tape, then sterilized. Verify appropriate color change has been achieved in external process indicator immediately after removal from sterilizer then check internal process indicator before treatment. Refer to state regulations for any additional state requirements.

One Ring and Arm Positioning System

Functions ▶ To position and hold digital sensors or film in patient's mouth for periapical and bite-wing images using parallel technique

To allow patient to bite on holder to keep digital sensor or film in place while positioning the position-indicating device (PID) and exposing the sensor or film

Reduces the number of components needed for positioning—one arm, one ring

Characteristics ▶
1 Holds film for bite-wing projection—barrier placed on sensor
2 Holds film for anterior and posterior teeth projections—barrier placed on sensor
3 Holds film for posterior teeth projection—barrier placed on sensor

Slots on ring are color coded—blue, anterior; yellow, posterior; red, bite-wing
Allows sufficient amount of space for sensors with wires

Practice Notes ▶ Uses the parallel technique for exposing radiation to the sensor or film
PID is parallel with the ring using a round or square PID

Sterilization Notes ▶ Disassembled Holders must be precleaned, either, placed in a sterilizing pouch with an internal process indicator, sealed, then sterilized OR wrapped with an internal process indicator inside and secured on the outside with process indicator tape, then sterilized. Verify appropriate color change has been achieved in external process indicator immediately after removal from sterilizer then check internal process indicator before treatment. Refer to state regulations for any additional state requirements.

Rinn XCP Holders for Digital Sensors

Functions ▶ To position and hold digital sensor in patient's mouth for periapical and bite-wing images, using parallel technique
To allow patient to bite on holder to keep sensor in place while positioning the position-indicating device (PID) and exposing the electronic sensor

Characteristics ▶
1 Blue—Holds film for anterior teeth projection
2 Red—Holds film for bite-wing projection
3 Yellow—Holds film for posterior teeth projection
4 Green—Holds film when taking projections for endodontic procedures

Slots hold electronic sensor in place with barriers placed on sensor and wire.

Practice Note ▶ Several different styles of electronic sensor holders are available.

Sterilization Notes ▶ Dissembled Holders must be precleaned, either, placed in a sterilizing pouch with an internal process indicator, sealed, then sterilized OR wrapped with an internal process indicator inside and secured on the outside with process indicator tape, then sterilized. Verify appropriate color change has been achieved in external process indicator immediately after removal from sterilizer then check internal process indicator before treatment. Refer to state regulations for any additional state requirements.

Digital Intraoral X-Ray Unit

Functions ▶ To take digital intraoral images without film or without processing the film
To project the image of the teeth by digitally projecting radiation onto an electronic sensor and then to computerized imaging system

Characteristics ▶
1 Position-indicating device (PID) (round)
2 Tube head
3 X-ray unit with digital panel
4 Rectangular PID

Digital radiographs use less radiation than conventional radiographs.
Networks to computers in all areas of the dental office
Immediate imaging available

Practice Notes ▶ Paperless dental offices store digital x-rays on the computer, along with patient records. Used in all phases of dentistry, especially endodontics, orthodontics, oral surgery, and implantology.

Sterilization Notes ▶ Follow standard precautions and cross contamination protocol when exposing and processing film. Barriers should be used on x-ray tube head, PID and panel where x-ray button is pushed. If barriers are not used follow manufacturer's recommendation for precleaning and disinfecting of the Dental X-Ray Unit. Refer to state regulations for any additional state requirements.

Portable X-Ray Unit

Functions ▶ To take intraoral images with a portable device
To expose digital sensors or conventional dental radiographic film

Characteristics ▶ Wide color LCD with easy to recognize preset exposure; preset exposure time can be adjusted with one button
Unit has a 3.0-mA current
Features internal shielding and a backscatter shield to ensure safety and minimize x-ray exposure to operator and patient
Can be used in place of wall-mounted units

Practice Notes ▶ The battery pack is separate from the body of the unit to minimize the weight and reduce stress on the operator's shoulders and arms.

Sterilization Notes ▶ Follow standard precautions and cross-contamination protocol when exposing and processing film. Barriers should be used on X-ray Unit. If not, follow manufacturer's recommendation for precleaning and disinfection of the Dental X-Ray Unit. Refer to state regulations for any additional state requirements.

SCANX Digital Imaging System

Function ▶ To produce diagnostic intraoral digital images

Characteristics ▶ Uses phosphor storage plates (PSPs)—Plastic plates coated with an x-ray sensitive phosphor material

Plates reused multiple times using one time only plastic barrier for each patient that covers the plates

Plates placed in machine to erase current image taken

Different size plates available for images

Compatible computer software needed for the SCANX digital images

Images appear on computer screen

Computer software compatibility of enhancing digital images to aid in diagnosis

Practice Note ▶ Use regular intraoral x-ray machines for images

Use requirements—SCANX, computer and practice management software

Can be used in normal room lighting

Sterilization Notes ▶ Follow standard precautions and cross-contamination protocol. Barriers must be used when exposing sensors. Each plastic plate is covered and closed with a plastic barrier. Plastic barrier is removed before placing in SCANX. New plastic barrier is used for each SCANX image. Plastic covers are one time use only and disposed of in garbage after each use. Refer to state regulations for any additional state requirements.

Extraoral X-Rays—Cephalometric and Panoramic

Functions ▶ To use to project the patient's teeth through x-ray onto the film
To use for extraoral projections

Characteristics ▶ Film is placed in a cassette outside the mouth.

1 Cephalometric radiograph—Shows bony and soft-tissue areas of the facial profile

2 Panoramic radiograph—Shows a panoramic view of maxillary and mandibular teeth on one film

Practice Notes ▶ Different styles of extraoral radiograph machines are available.
Cephalometric and panoramic digital radiographs
Cephalometric and panoramic radiographs are used in all phases of dentistry. Panoramic images are used frequently in orthodontics.

Sterilization Notes ▶ Follow standard precautions and cross-contamination protocol when exposing and processing film for developing.

▪INSTRUMENT Digital Panoramic/Cephalometric Imaging Unit

Functions ▶ To take digital panoramic and cephalometric images without film or without processing the film

To project the image of maxillary and mandibular teeth by digitally projecting radiation onto an electronic sensor and then to computerized imaging system

Characteristics ▶ Unit pictured is a 3 in 1 unit that takes both panoramic and cephalometic images. (It also takes 3D CBCT scans.)

Digital radiographs use less radiation than conventional radiographs.

Networks to computers in all areas of the dental office

Immediate imaging available

Practice Notes ▶ Paperless dental offices store digital panoramic imaging on the computer, along with patient records.

Used in all phases of dentistry, especially orthodontics, oral surgery, and implantology. Panoramic and cephalometric images may also be taken with conventional film.

Sterilization Notes ▶ Follow standard precautions and cross-contamination protocol. Barriers should be used, if not, then, follow the manufacturer's recommendation for precleaning and disinfection.

Cone-Beam Three-Dimensional (3D) Imaging System

Function ▶ To produce diagnostic 3D images of the head and neck as related to dentistry

Characteristics ▶ High-resolution scans produce images at 0.2-mm voxel size to provide diagnosis for difficult areas to view with conventional radiographs.

Typical scan time of 8.9 seconds

Less radiation and more comfortable for the patient

Practice Note ▶ Assists in diagnosis for enhanced orthodontic treatment planning, supernumerary teeth, abnormal anomalies, third molars, small root fractures, periodontal conditions, relationship of dentition, and other anatomy requiring detailed visualization

Sterilization Notes ▶ Follow standard precautions and cross-contamination protocol. Barriers should be used, if not, then, follow the manufacturer's recommendation for precleaning and disinfection.

Examination under incandescent light

Biopsy-confirmed oral cancer

Using the VELscope Vx

Enhanced Oral Assessment System—VELscope Vx

Function ▶ To aid in the assessment of oral mucosal abnormalities in early visualization of potential oral cancer, precancerous lesions or tissue, infections, and trauma that are not apparent to the naked eye alone

To use as an aid in determining surgical boundaries of oral lesions for excision

To use in conjunction with the traditional intraoral and extraoral examination. Referred to as the comprehensive oral exam (COE)

Characteristics ▶ Technology is based on an imaging modality that is sensitive to tissue changes that illuminates oral cavity to visualize potential abnormalities.

Handheld device emits a harmless, ultraviolet (UV) light used to inspect the oral cavity.

Device is sensitive to abnormal tissue changes. Distinctive blue-spectrum light causes the soft tissue (oral mucosa) of the mouth to naturally fluoresce.

Imaging adapter with iPod touch attaches to VELscope Vx eyepiece for clinical photographic documentation

Practice Note ▶ Velscope Vx is implemented in general practice as well as periodontal and maxillofacial surgery practices.

Sterilization Notes ▶ Protective barriers should be used on the device for each patient such as VELcap Vx and VELsheath Vx, which is recommended for each patient examination. Manufacturer's recommendation should be followed for precleaning and disinfecting the unit.

Vital Signs and Beyond

Stethoscope

Functions ▶ To listen to pulse
To listen to heartbeat
To listen to systolic and diastolic pressure when taking blood pressure

Characteristics ▶
1. Ear pieces to hear pulse, and/or blood pressure
2. Device to place on an artery to hear the sounds from the pulse, systolic and diastolic pressure Usually, blood pressure is taken at the brachial artery in the arm.

Practice Notes ▶ Stethoscope in dentistry is used in conjunction with blood pressure cuff to hear systolic and diastolic pressure.
Stethoscope is used before dental procedures to hear the pulse, and take blood pressure

Sterilization Notes ▶ Stethoscope should be precleaned and disinfected according to the manufacturer's recommendation.

Aneroid Blood Pressure Cuff—Sphygmomanometer

Functions ▶ To place pressure on the arteries to hear the systolic and diastolic pressure of the arteries

To place around the part of the arm above the bend in the elbow

Characteristics ▶
1. Blood pressure cuff for the arm
2. Meter—Aneroid dial system (without liquid); the readout for systolic and diastolic blood pressure
3. Rubber bulb—Attached to cuff with rubber tubing

Blood pressure cuff available in regular size, small size, and larger size cuffs to fit various arm sizes

Cuff size should fit properly to obtain accurate blood pressure readings.

Cuff is placed above the bend in the elbow above the brachial artery.

Practice Notes ▶ Blood Pressure Cuff is used in conjunction with the stethoscope to hear the systolic and diastolic pressure at the brachial artery located at the inner side of the bend in the elbow.

Document blood pressure readings in patient's chart.

Sterilization Notes ▶ Blood Pressure Cuff must be precleaned and disinfected according to the manufacturer's recommendation.

Automatic Blood Pressure Monitor

Functions ▶ To measure blood pressure automatically
To display the blood pressure readout on the screen
To measure pulse rate automatically
To display the pulse readout on the screen

Characteristics ▶ Blood pressure cuff
Readout screen for blood pressure and pulse rate

Blood pressure cuff available in regular size, small size,
and larger size cuffs to fit various arms
Correct cuff size important for accurate blood pressure
readings
Data from past blood pressure information available on some monitors

Practice Notes ▶ Automatic Blood Pressure Monitor is used before medical and dental procedures.
Document blood pressure readings in patient's chart.

Sterilization Notes ▶ Blood Pressure Cuff must be precleaned and disinfected according to the manufacturer's
recommendation.

Electrocardiogram (EKG) Machine

Function ▶ To measure the electrical activity of the heartbeat

Characteristics ▶ EKG chest leads; self-adhesive pads with wires attached with electrodes for conductivity and placed in specific locations on the patient which are connected to the EKG machine
A read-out is displayed on the screen.

Practice Note ▶ EKG Machine is used to monitor the patient's heartbeat usually during dental surgical procedures, during intravenous sedation in a dental office (mostly for oral surgeries), and for general anesthesia.

Sterilization Notes ▶ Chest leads are single use only. Chest leads used on the patient are disposable and should be disposed of in garbage. Single use only. Disinfect unit according to manufacturer's recommendation.

▪INSTRUMENT Pulse Oximeter

Functions ▶ To measure the concentration of oxygen in the blood
To detect the pulse rate

Characteristics ▶
1. Monitor to display oxygen concentration in the blood and pulse rate
2. Finger device that measures the oxygen concentration and pulse rate that sends information to the monitor

Practice Note ▶ Pulse Oximetry used to monitor the patient's heart beat as well as oxygen concentration usually during dental surgical procedures, during intravenous sedation in a dental office, and for general anesthesia

Sterilization Notes ▶ Pulse Oximetry should be precleaned and disinfected according to the manufacturer's recommendation.

Capnograph

Functions ▶ To measure carbon dioxide (CO_2) in exhaled breath
To monitor patient's ventilation

Characteristics ▶
1 Capnograph monitors patient ventilation, providing a breath by breath trend of respirations and an early warning system of impending respiratory crisis.
2 Monitor displays patient carbon dioxide in exhaled breath.

Capnography provides an immediate picture of patient condition.
Example: Holding your breath. Capnograph will show immediate apnea. Pulse oximetry is delayed for several minutes, and the pulse oximeter will show high saturation of oxygen for several minutes with holding your breath.

When a person hyperventilates, their CO_2 decreases.

Practice Note ▶ Used in dental offices for patients who are sedated

Sterilization Notes ▶ Capnograph should be precleaned and disinfected according to the manufacturer's recommendations.

Automated External Defibrillator (AED)

Functions ▶ To use for emergency situations when a person is unresponsive
To use when a person has no pulse and is not breathing

Characteristic ▶ Place devices correctly on patient and wait
for automated voice directions from AED to
proceed.

Practice Notes ▶ A provider should be trained healthcare provider
basic life support along with using an AED.
Preventive maintenance is required for update
of batteries.

Sterilization Notes ▶ AED should be precleaned and disinfected
according to the manufacturer's recommendations.

Index

Note: Page numbers followed by *f* indicate figures.